THE SIRT DIET COOKBOOK

THE BEST COOKBOOK WITH SIRT DIET RECIPES TO LOSE WEIGHT, BURN FAT, AND ACTIVATE YOUR METABOLISM. FOLLOW THESE HEALTHY RECIPES TO IMPROVE YOUR LIFESTYLE.

Emily Baker

TABLE OF CONTENTS

INTRODUCTION 7

CHAPTER 1 9

WHAT IS SIRT FOOD? 9

CHAPTER 2 11

THE SCIENCE OF SIRTUINS 11

CHAPTER 3

THE REASONS WHY THE SIRT DIET IS SUITABLE 17

CHAPTER 4 FOOD LIST 21

CHAPTER 5

 WHAT ARE THE STEPS TO APPLY THE DIET? 25

CHAPTER 6 SIRTFOOD AROUND THE WORLD 31

CHAPTER 7 RECIPES 35

BREAKFAST 35

KALE AND BLACKCURRANT SMOOTHIE 36

CHOCOLATE CUPCAKES WITH MATCHA ICING 37

GREEN TEA SMOOTHIE 38

TURMERIC CHICKEN & KALE SALAD

 WITH HONEY-LIME 39

BAKED SALMON SALAD WITH CREAMY MINT 40

COQ AU VIN 41

KALE WHITE BEAN PORK SOUP 42

TURKEY SATAY SKEWERS 43

TOMATO & GOAT'S CHEESE PIZZA 44

TOFU THAI CURRY 45

TOMATO & GOAT'S CHEESE PIZZA 46

KALE WALNUT BAKE 47

KALE-GREEN BEAN CASSEROLE 48

RICE WITH LEMON AND ARUGULA 49

CAJUN TURKEY STUFFING 50

PURPLE POTATOES WITH ONIONS,

MUSHROOMS, AND CAPERS 51

CAJUN TURKEY STUFFING 52

KING PRAWN STIR-FRY

WITH BUCKWHEAT NOODLES 53

PRAWN & CHILI PAK CHOI 54

PRAWN & CHILI PAK CHOI 55

SMOKED SALMON OMELET 56

MUSSELS IN RED WINE SAUCE 57

GINGER PRAWN STIR-FRY 58

TURKEY MOLE TACOS 59

CHICKEN WITH BALSAMIC ONIONS

AND MUSHROOMS 60

CHICKEN & BEAN CASSEROLE 61

CHICKEN CURRY WITH POTATOES AND KALE 62

SPINACH AND TURKEY LASAGNA 63

TENDER SPICED LAMB 64

STEAK & MUSHROOM NOODLES 65

ROAST LAMB & RED WINE SAUCE 66

SIRTFOOD CAULIFLOWER

COUSCOUS & TURKEY STEAK 67

TURKEY CURRY 68

FRIED CAULIFLOWER RICE 69

VEGETARIAN CURRY FROM THE CROCK-POT 70

MEXICAN BELL PEPPER FILLED WITH EGG: 71

FRITTATA WITH SPRING ONIONS

AND ASPARAGUS: 72

VEGETARIAN PALEO RATATOUILLE: 73

LENTIL & GREENS SOUP CORN

AND BLACK BEAN SOUP   74

BUCKWHEAT SPLIT PEA SOUP   75

HOT AND SOUR MISO SOUP   76

GARLIC, SPINACH, AND CHICKPEA SOUP   77

CAJUN SHRIMP SOUP   78

EXOTIC MUESLI WITH TROPICAL FRUITS   79

SPICY MANGO SALAD WITH SHEEP'S CHEESE   80

CLOUD BREAD   81

CUCUMBER AND PINEAPPLE SALAD

WITH MACKEREL   82

SALAD WITH EGG, RADICCHIO

AND POTATO PASTE   83

STRAWBERRY BUCKWHEAT PANCAKES   84

PANCAKES WITH APPLES AND BLACKCURRANTS   85

RAW VEGAN WALNUTS PIE CRUST

& RAW BROWNIES   86

PALEO CHOCOLATE WRAPS WITH FRUITS   87

CHOCOLATE GRANOLA   88

CONCLUSION   92

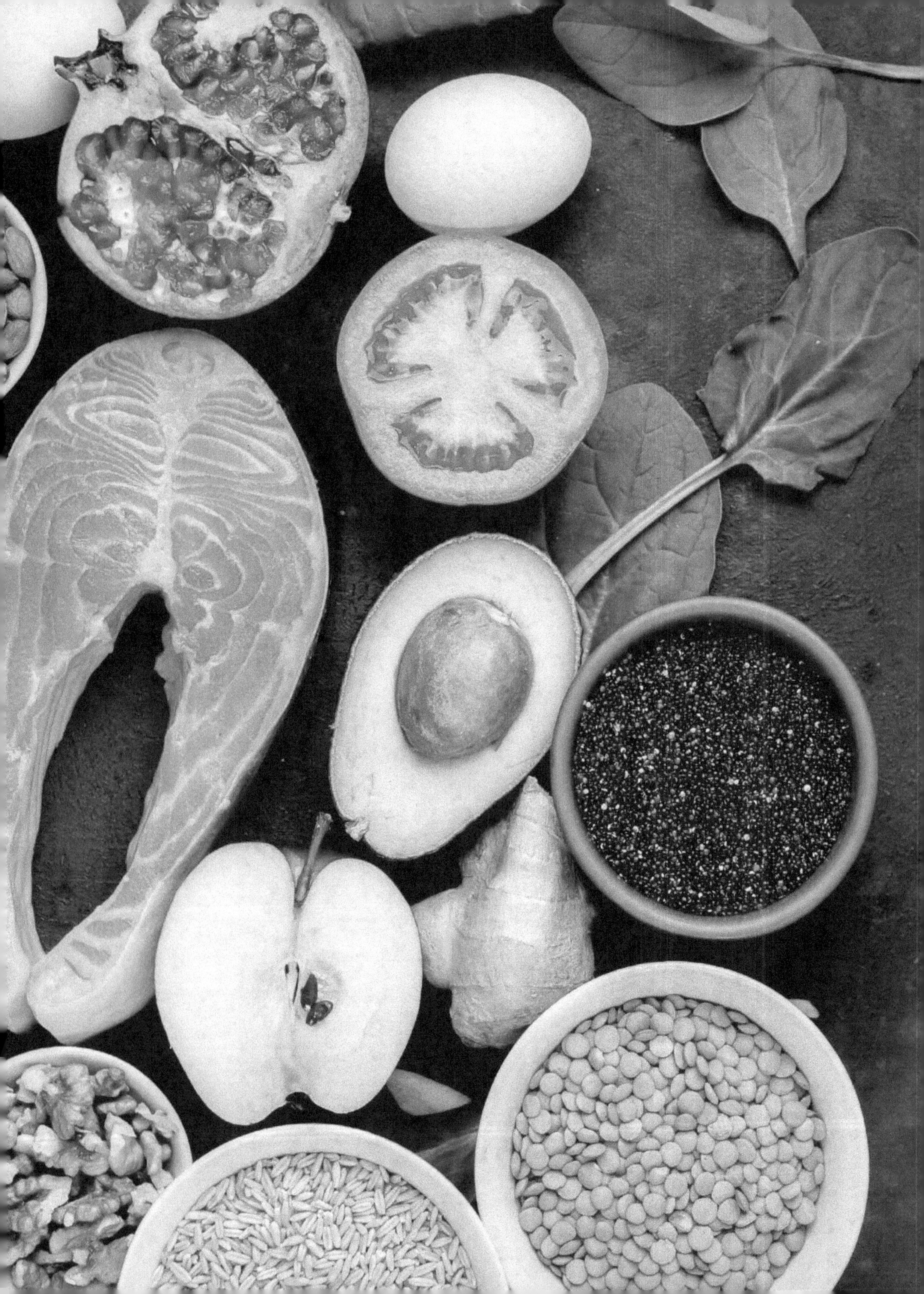

INTRODUCTION

Let us get one thing straight! Sirtuins were discovered many years ago, but the SirtFoods diet came to light in 2003 in a groundbreaking study when it was discovered by researchers that resveratrol, a compound found in red wine and red-grape skin, significantly increase the lifecycle of yeast. Generally, there are many researches that need to be carried out before we can fully understand all the benefits of this diet. So far, through research, people are getting to understand the full benefits of these high foods, majorly foods already enjoyed, from strawberries to red wine or cocoa. The natural components of these foods have the ability to mimic skinny genes" in our bodies as fasting and exercise does; they can also suppress appetite and build muscle. There is no argument whatsoever about the health benefits of eating fruits and vegetables; they are a great source of rich vitamins, minerals, and protein.

In contrast, there is a clash of opinion as a few people still believe they cannot get all the required protein to maintain the muscle mass from just plants, hereby embracing meats and fish into their meal; without any need to argue that fruits and vegetables are a good source of protein. However, following a sirtfood diet does not mean you can only eat foods that are highly sirtuin concentrated or automatically make you a vegetarian. Eating meat, fish, milk, cheese, eggs, etc. are other suitable sources of getting enough protein in your body. The sirtfood diet does not forbid you from enjoying the food you love to eat; in fact, no food is left behind. The idea is eating healthy by reducing some harmful foods like high carb or processed foods and replacing them with more of sirtuin foods. One of the disadvantages of carb is the constant cravings; by substituting high carb food with these particular kinds of protein, you can put an end to carb craving, you will no longer feel hungry as you used to because sirtfood diet naturally suppresses your craving. Appetite suppression and calorie deprivation will lead to weight loss, your insulin level will drop, your blood sugar level will reduce, and you will feel healthier and more alive. A proper diet should not only focus on weight loss and neglect the overall health. It is pointless to follow a diet that makes you lose weight rapidly but jeopardize your overall health. The sirt diet will help you lower blood sugar level and drop insulin level, so you do not need to worry about most health problems like inflammation, diabetes, cancer, etc., which are all caused by poor nutrition.

Now, you have a reason to embrace the sirtfood diet, set a long term goal, and make sirt food a lifestyle.

Do not know what to eat? You will find plenty of sirtfood recipes here to help you get started and stay on course.

CHAPTER 1
WHAT IS SIRT FOOD?

It's a small revolution in the world of nutrition. Its name is already in everyone's mouths across the Channel: "The Sirt food diet" promises to convince the most resistant to diets because this one is not like the others. No question of depriving yourself, but rather of adding elements to your diet.

The principle is simple: bet everything on "superfoods," such as apples, onions, green tea … or dark chocolate and red wine. These are natural activators of the sirtuin enzymes present in our body, themselves endowed with the capacity to stimulate the "discomfort of thinness." Aidan Goggins and Glen Matten define themselves as " nutrition geeks, "and can boast of the support of British sportsmen and top models. Their diet would be able to make you lose 7 pounds in 7 days (about 3 kgs).

This diet comes from England, and, more precisely, from two nutritionists: Aidan Goggins and Glen Matten. Their objective? Eat healthily rather than lose weight at all costs, because, unlike other diets programmed to lose weight, even unhealthy drastically, the Sirt Food diet rather wants to stimulate the immune system, while eliminating fat. Besides, the Sirtfood diet would be able to make you lose 3 pounds in 7 days, without any deprivation.

By favoring sirt foods, this diet aims to improve your mode of consumption. Among these greedy "elected," there are many fruits and vegetables such as apples, citrus fruits, strawberries, kale but also parsley, red onion, capers, green tea, soy, turmeric, olive oil, coffee and, more surprisingly, red wine and chocolate (dark of course)! For the most suspicious, know that the countries where people eat the most sirt foods (Japan and Italy) are ranked among the healthiest in the world.

It authorizes the consumption

of foods that are prohibited in most other slimming diets, including, in particular, chocolate and red wine. If its creators are to be believed, it will allow, despite this, to lose up to 3 kg in the space of 7 days without really depriving yourself. Here we give you the typical menu for this diet which has already won over more than one.

The typical menu

Here is an example of a typical sirtfood day menu:

- At breakfast: soy yogurt mixed with berries, chopped nuts, and dark chocolate. If you prefer to opt for salty, start the day with a bacon omelet accompanied by red chicory and parsley.

- At lunch: a sirtfood salad (chicory leaves, avocado, lovage, capers, etc.) will do the trick. But you can also replace it with a pita garnished with cheese, hummus, and turkey.

- At dinner: sautéed shrimps with buckwheat noodles and kale. You can also opt for a homemade pizza made with sirtfood foods.

During the first three days of the diet, it is advisable to limit yourself to 1000 calories per day by drinking three green juices made from foods rich in sirtuins. From the 4th to the 7th day, the diet allows you to bring your daily caloric consumption to 1500 calories always by including in large quantities foods rich in sirtuins in the preparation of these meals.

This amounts to taking two sirtfood smoothies and two meals rich in sirtuins per day. Finally, from the 8th day, you must find a balanced daily diet while maintaining sirtfood in your meals.

Slimming without really depriving yourself with sirtuins

The sirtfood diet is based on the principle that consuming foods rich in sirtuins is enough to lose weight without actually having to deprive yourself. Sirtuins are proteins naturally synthesized by the body, which increase the body's ability to burn fat, activate the metabolism, and consolidate muscle mass. They also have an anti-aging effect.

They can be found in around twenty fairly common foods, including red wine, dark chocolate, apples, soy, dates, buckwheat, parsley, arugula, spinach, celery, capers, l olive oil, green tea, etc.

The sirtfood diet is very attractive because it allows you to lose weight without suffering too much by adopting a French menu simple and easy to carry out. However, like all weight loss programs of this type, this diet presents relatively significant risks, especially if it is prolonged beyond the first seven days.

CHAPTER 2
THE SCIENCE OF SIRTUINS

The basis of the sirtuin diet can be explained in simple terms or complex ways. It is important to understand how and why it works, however, so that you can appreciate the value of what you are doing. It is important also to know why these sirtuin rich foods help to help you maintain fidelity to your diet plan. Otherwise, you may throw something in your meal with less nutrition that would defeat the purpose of planning for one rich in sirtuins. Most importantly, this is not a dietary fad, and as you will see, there is much wisdom contained in how humans have used natural foods even for medicinal purposes, over thousands of years.

To understand how the Sirtfood diet works, and why these particular foods are necessary, we will look at the role they play in the human body.

Sirtuin activity was first researched in yeast, where a mutation caused an extension in the yeast's lifespan. Sirtuins were also shown to slow aging in laboratory mice, fruit flies, and nematodes. As research on Sirtuins proved to transfer to mammals, they were examined for their use in diet and slowing the aging process. The sirtuins in humans are different in typing, but they essentially work in the same ways and reasons.

There are seven "members" that make up the sirtuin family. It is believed that sirtuins play a big role in regulating certain functions of cells, including proliferation (reproduction and growth of cells), apoptosis (death of cells). They promote survival and resist stress to increase longevity.

They are also seen to block neurodegeneration (loss of function of the nerve cells in the brain). They conduct their housekeeping functions by cleaning out toxic proteins and supporting the brain's ability to change and adapt to different conditions, or to recuperate (i.e., brain plasticity). As part of this, they also help reduce chronic inflammation and reduce something called oxidative stress. Oxidative stress is when there are too many cell-damaging free radicals circulating in the body, and the body cannot catch up by combating them with anti-oxidants. These factors are related to age-related illness and weight as well, which again, brings us back to a discussion of how they work.

You will see labels in Sirtuins that start with "SIR," which represents "Silence Information Regulator" genes. They do exactly that, silence or regulate, as part of their functions. The seven sirtuins that humans work with are SIRT1, SIRT2, SIRT3, SIRT4, SIRT 5, SIRT6, and SIRT7. Each of these types is responsible for different areas of protecting cells. They work by either stimulating or turning on certain gene expressions, or by reducing and turning off other gene expressions. This essentially means that they can influence genes to do more or less of something, most of which they are already programmed to do.

Through enzyme reactions, each of the SIRT types affects different areas of cells that are responsible for the metabolic processes that help to maintain life. This is also related to what organs and functions they will affect.

For example, the expression of the SIRT6 cause of genes in humans that affect skeletal muscle, fat tissue, brain, and heart. SIRT 3 would cause the expression of genes that affect the kidneys, liver, brain, and heart.

If we tie these concepts together, you can see that the Sirtuin proteins can change the expression of genes, and in the case of the Sirtfood Diet, we care about how sirtuins can turn off those genes that are responsible for speeding up aging and for weight management.

The other aspect to this conversation of sirtuins is the function and the power of calorie restriction on the human body. Calorie restriction is simply eating fewer calories. This, coupled with exercise and reducing stress, is usually a combination of weight loss. Calorie restriction has also proven across much research in animals and humans to increase one's lifespan.

We can look further at the role of sirtuins with calorie restriction and using the SIRT3 protein, which has a role in metabolism and aging. Amongst all of the effects of the protein on gene expression (such as preventing cells from dying, reducing tumors from growing, etc.), we want to understand the effects of SIRT3 on weight.

The SIRT3 has high expression in those metabolically active tissues, as we stated earlier, and its ability to express itself increases with caloric restriction, fasting, and exercise. On the contrary, it will express itself less when the body has high fat, high calorie-riddled diet.

The last few highlights of sirtuins are their role in regulating telomeres and reducing inflammation, which also helps with staving off disease and aging.

Telomeres are sequences of proteins at the ends of chromosomes. When cells divide, these get shorter. As we age, they get shorter, and other stressors to the body also will contribute to this. Maintaining these longer telomeres is the key to slower aging. Also, proper diet, along with exercise and other variables, can lengthen telomeres. SIRT6 is one of the sirtuins that, if activated, can help with DNA damage, inflammation, and oxidative stress. SIRT1 also helps with inflammatory response cycles that are related to many age-related diseases.

Calories restriction, as we mentioned earlier, can extend life to some degree.

Since this, as well as fasting, is a stressor, these factors will stimulate the SIRT3 proteins to kick in and protect the body from the stressors and excess free radicals. Again, the telomere length is affected as well.

To sum up, all of this information also shows that, contrary to some people's beliefs that in terms of genetics, such as "it is what it is" or "it is my fate because Uncle Joe has something…" through our own lifestyle choices. What we are exposed to, we can influence action and changes in our genes. This is quite an empowering thought and yet another reason why you should be excited to have a science-based diet such as the Sirtfood diet, available to you.

Having laid this all out before you, you should be able to appreciate how and why these miraculous compounds work in your favor to keep you youthful, healthy, and lean If they are working hard for you, don't you feel that you should do something too?

Sirtfood diet refers to foods that are aimed at losing calories by activating your skinny gene known as sirtuins. Sirtuins play a key role in regulating homeostasis, which involves keeping the cell in balance. SIRTs are a group of seven proteins in the body that regulate a variety of functions such as lifespan, metabolism, and inflammation. Certain foods are believed to increase the level of these proteins in the body, therefore, being referred to as sirtfoods.

These sirtfoods include:

- dark chocolate-at least 85% cocoa

- red chicory capers

- kale arugula blueberries walnut

- red wine strawberries turmeric apples

- soy parsley green tea

- red onions buckwheat citrus fruits

- coffee Medjool dates cinnamon

The sirtfoods contain a chemical called polyphenols that have the same effects as exercising and fasting. The diet combines sirtfoods and calorie restriction, leading to higher sirtuin production levels. Sirtuin foods deprive the energy of the body, making it to use glycogen, leading to the burning of fat and muscle gain. Each glycogen molecule requires 3-4 water molecules.

Sirtuins are a group of seven proteins that maintain cell metabolism and homeostasis at optimal levels. Three of these proteins are found in the mitochondria, one is in the cytoplasm, and another three are located in the nucleus. Sirtuins maintain the health of the cell and ensure that all processes going on within the cell are properly happening. Sirtuins can, however, not be effective without the presence of NAD+ (nicotinamide adenine dinucleotide). NAD+ is a coenzyme that is present in all cells that are living in nature. NAD+ ensures that Sirtuins function optimally and can regulate cells.

Homeostasis within the cell is the process of maintaining all the numerous functions of the cell at stability, which ensures balance. It may also involve the maintenance of PH, and the saturate concentration levels of the cytoplasm, which is the most significant component of the cell in terms of volume. All these are aspects of the cell that must stay constant for optimal cell health. Sirtuins perform several functions, among them being the ability to deacetylase proteins called histones. Acetyls are proteins with a physical form of Histones are proteins that contain a condensed form of DNA called chromatins, which prevent the proteins from performing their functions in this acetyl.

The deacetylation, therefore, frees the proteins for the undertaking of their respective functions, given that proteins are the building blocks for the body. Proteins are proverbially referred to as bodybuilding foods. Without Sirtuins, therefore, the bodybuilding foods would fail to build our bodies as they are the critical components for freeing the protein molecules in our cells for their functions.

Role of Sirtuins in weight Loss

The Sirtuins are the CEO of a company, while the NAD+ is the financial resources that enable the company to pay the salaries of the CEO and the staff. The coenzyme NAD+, therefore, creates a medium for all cell activities to take place. Still, the Sirtuins are responsible for the regulation of all the cell activities, ensuring what needs to happen chances, and appropriately so. This means that NAD+ is the finances that pay for all the salaries and bills such as the lights and the rent of the premises for the firm. At the same time, the Sirtuins are the CEO, which ensures that every worker is at their station and doing what they are supposed to do, correctly and efficiently.

Workers in an office are supposed to do their work efficiently and effectively for as long as possible without fail. Sirtuins, therefore, also ensure optimal cell health, is maintained for as long as possible without fail. Sirtuins are therefore sought of the inhibiting factors preventing the cell from going overboard and malfunctioning (Health, 2015). Sirtuins' role in the cell, therefore, avoid cavities from bursting or from shrinking by maintaining the right PH the concentration and saturation levels of the cell cytoplasm and so forth. It is, however, eminent that the NAD+ coenzyme does not stay at optimum levels long enough throughout the life cycle of a person.

As people get older, therefore, NAD+ levels diminish, creating an imbalance in optimal cell health. The diminishing levels of the coenzyme could, therefore, be the reason why cells may become cancerous, for example. In older people, many cell processes fail, leading them to sicknesses they did not expect due to their cell activity being extremely compromised due to malfunctions caused by low NAD+

levels. Although it is not entirely understood why older people become more prone to certain illnesses, the study of Sirtuins and how they work is very critical in the beginning to understand the phenomena. The research, therefore, is still needed in the topic.

Understanding exactly what occurs after the diminishing levels of the NAD+ coenzyme could shed light on science as to just what causes such diseases as cancer, which are a considerable threat to human health and could wipe out the human race. Other chronic illnesses that may be caused by cell health deterioration are such as Alzheimer's disease, which is caused by the decline and death of brain cells of the human brain. A loss in cognitive abilities is a common symptom of the disease, which has no cure up to this very date.

CHAPTER 3 THE REASONS WHY THE SIRT DIET IS SUITABLE

In our diet, members lost 7 pounds in the underlying seven days, reminiscent of increased muscle and muscle work. This emotional impact on fat consumption as muscles grows one of the reasons why our sirt food diet has become so common to all those who lose weight and how to get in shape. World-class competitors and the models they make have supported this direction like a violin. Sirtfoods not only consume fat but also have the extraordinary ability to satisfy hunger. This makes it the ideal answer to reach a solid weight and last a long time.

However, considering it absolutely as dieting means ignoring the main problem. It's a diet that has as much to do with health as it does with size. Increased vitality, clearer skin, a progressive alarm, and better rest are the delicious "symptoms" of these power lines. Sometimes the benefits are more and more exceptional, recalling the situations where a longer diet has modified metabolic disorders. These are the effects that improve your well-being, and critics show that they are more dominant than drugs that are taken care of by doctors to prevent long-term illness, with benefits for diabetes, coronary artery disease, and disease. Alzheimer's disease, to name a few.

The main concern is clear: if you want to get an increasingly hot, less fatty, and more beneficial body and you want to create the framework for lifetime well-being and protection against diseases, the Sirtfood diet is made for you.

Here at the International Food Information Council Foundation, we are moving away from fad diets. For the most part, we reveal them and promote a fair food deal with room for guilty joys and vacations. Sometimes the diets we are talking about depend on certain strict livelihood rules and others that we cannot accept exist. This next diet, which we are going to talk about, falls into the last class. The newest addition to the diet scene is the sort of food diet, and we're here to show you why you don't have to face this kind of limitation in your life - it's neither scientific nor practical.

The positive effects of the SirtFood diet are listed below so that you can define your expectations and better understand the beautiful effects of the SirtFood diet (you can see the full view once the diet is started).

- All of course- The SirtFood diet promotes the consumption of all-natural foods. In the SirtFood diet, most of the recommended foods are vegetables. This means that your body is also detoxified by harmful chemicals, processed foods, and junk food.

- Burns fat and suppresses appetite- As explained above, the reason why this diet caresses or activates your sirtuin. As a result, the fat is burned, and the appetite is suppressed. Also, SirtFood offers a selection of foods that can further promote fat burning when consumed, as sirtuins control the genes responsible for your fat and sugar.

- Increases overall health - Weight loss can certainly reduce the risk of various diseases. The selection of foods is naturally rich in nutrients and helps eliminate free radical damage. An example is green tea with its catechin component, which can fight cancer cells.

- It helps improve memory.- Good news for those who have bad memories of work or who wish to improve their memory. This diet is for you. Studies have shown that this diet can improve memory based on food intake. For example, consuming cocoa (rich in epicatechin, another activator of sirtuin) and one gram of turmeric can improve memory if consumed regularly.

- Acts as an antioxidant - This is mainly because the diet is rich in plant-based and fruit-based foods, which are known to cleanse the body and remove toxins.

- Helps control blood sugar. - The participants in the study of this diet showed remarkable improvements not only in their body fat rate but also in their blood sugar. This, in turn, is due to the selection of healthy foods. Eating sirtuin in apples and onions helps control the level of glucose in the body. Other sirtuin triggers can help regulate your sugar. Imagine that you combine these types of food and eat them regularly. This leads to a healthier change in your body.

- Very easy to follow- The SirtFood diet is flexible. Aside from consuming SirtFoods, there are no hard and fast rules. You can eat it yourself, add it to your regular meals, or find and consume concentrated versions of the recommended SirtFood. Also, no special dietary supplement or expensive food is required.

- No need for strenuous exercise or hunger- Although exercise is recommended, strenuous exercise is not necessary (unless you want to try it) because your body not only ingests healthier foods but also benefits from your "lean" gene. One thing that is guaranteed with this diet is that no fasting or hunger is required even during the first three days of the diet. You just need to make sure you plan and balance your calorie intake.

- Delays the anti-aging process - Sirtuins are actually "guardians" of the body's enzymes, which not only help protect cells but can also slow the aging process.

- It can fight inflammation. - Due to the powerful antioxidants in the diet, it can help fight inflammation in the body and protect the heart.

- No rebound effect - The SirtFood diet can promote rapid weight loss, especially in the first week. But don't worry, all the fat you've lost won't come back during the maintenance phase. There are no calorie control traps in this diet. With the SirtFood diet, your targeted sirtuins stimulate your system to burn fat and use excess glucose to build muscle. This means that no fat is stored.

In general, the SirtFood diet is effective and safe. There are only a few "drawbacks":

Weight loss in the pan- It can happen with any weight loss. It is a condition in which you actively participate in your weight loss program, but the balance does not seem to move. Check your food journal, intake, or try other foods full of sirtuin. You can also extend your exercise time by a few minutes (if available) to further increase your weight loss. While this is generally not a bad thing, you just need to find the right combination of foods. Be alarmed if you suddenly gain weight as it means something is wrong with your diet.

You should always check your general eating habits- If you add foods filled with sirtuin to each meal but continue to eat junk food or these low-calorie foods daily, you should not expect the scales to produce positive results.

Not too much material available.- Since the diet is relatively new, you may find few resources to gain additional knowledge about the diet. However, there is "enough" material, studies and testimonials to support your SirtFood journey.

Limits- Proponents of this diet make sure that you are not hungry with this nutritional program as long as you balance your decisions. But yes, the first week with the 1000/1500 limitation can be stressful. But as we say, there is no gain without pain! You can certainly do it.

If you already have an illness, consult your doctor before trying this diet. Please note that this diet is not suitable for pregnant women who want to keep their weight or women who are trying to conceive.

Before starting a diet, you should try to weigh the pros and cons. In addition to guaranteed weight loss, the SirtFood diet offers many health benefits. For the downsides, it means accepting the challenge and making the necessary efforts to overcome it. When you've made your decision, take that first step and start the diet!

The SirtFood diet is suitable for people who:

1. Are overweight or obese

2. You want to keep your weight.

3. You must have a "detoxification" and eliminate toxins from your body.

4. You have failed to lose weight with various eating techniques.

5. You want to lose not only weight but also build muscle.

6. They want a healthier lifestyle and optimal health.

CHAPTER 4
FOOD LIST

Arugula

This green salad leaf (also known as rucola) is very common in the Mediterranean diet. It is not too popular in the US food culture, and it is considered an absolute arrogance to have it on your plate. However, we're not talking about a leaf covered in gold or silver; we're talking about a green salad leaf with a peppery taste that can be used for digestive and diuretic purposes. During the time of ancient Rome and in the Middle Ages, this leaf was known to have aphrodisiac properties. However, there's a lot more to this miracle leaf. It has nutrients like quercetin and kaempferol capable of activating sirtuins. This combination is said to have very positive effects on the skin as it can moisturize and improve collagen synthesis. So why not have this leaf in your salad and add some extra olive oil on it, making it a powerful sirtfood duo? As you can see, it has a lot of positive effects on your body.

Buckwheat

This is one of the best sources for rutin, a sirtuin-activator nutrient. However, this crop is also amazing for ecological and sustainable farming, as it can improve the quality of the soil and prevent weed growth. However, probably the most interesting part about buckwheat is that it is a fruit seed, kind of like rhubarb, so it is not a grain at all. There isn't a coincidence at all that buckwheat has more protein than any grain known to man, so it fits perfectly in your sirtfood diet. For every person trying to avoid gluten, this can be the ideal food. It is the ideal alternative for grains.

Capers

Some of you may not be too familiar with capers. If you haven't had the chance to taste them, you should. They are those dark-green salty things you can sometimes see on top of a pizza. Unfortunately, capers are not very used in a standard diet (it is very overlooked and underrated), but those who never had the chance to try capers don't know what they are missing. We are talking about the flower buds of the caper bush, a plant growing abundantly in the Mediterranean region. It is usually handpicked and preserved, and it has some interesting antidiabetic, anti-inflammatory, antimicrobial, antiviral, and immunomodulatory properties. Moreover, it has been used in medicine all around the Mediterranean area.

Capers are also rich in sirtuin-activating nutrients, so they have the chance to shine in the sirtfood diet, and I can guarantee that you will fall in love with them.

Celery

This is a plant used for thousands of years, as in ancient Egypt, people were already aware of it and its properties. Back then, it was considered a medicinal plant that can be used for detoxing, cleansing and preventing diseases. Therefore, celery consumption is very good for your gut, kidney, and liver. When it was growing wildly in ancient times, it had a strong bitter flavor. However, ever since its domestication in the 17th century, celery has become a bit sweeter, and now it can be used in salads.

There are two types of celery: Pascal (green) and blanched (yellow). Blanching is the technique used to reduce celery's bitter taste (too strong by many standards) by shading the plant from sunlight before harvesting. This leads to a milder flavor and a paler color. Unfortunately, the blanched celery is not the version you want if you want to reap the full benefits of this plant.

Luckily, the trend is changing, and more and more people are willing to try the green celery even though its taste is very bitter. This is the type I would recommend, as it contains plenty of nutrients to activate sirtuins. It may have a bitter taste, but you can use it in salads and green juices as well. Keep in mind that the most nutritious parts are the leaves and the hearts.

Chilies

This veggie should be in your diet, whether you like eating spicy food or not. It contains capsaicin, and this substance makes us savor it even more. Consuming chilies is great for activating sirtuins, and it speeds up your metabolism. The spicier the chili is, the more powerful it is when it comes to activating sirtuins. You probably heard that people eating spicy food three or four times per week have a 14 percent lower death rate compared to people who eat them less than once a week. Now, this doesn't mean that you have to go for the hottest chilies you can find, especially if you are not a spicy food enthusiast. Take it easy at the beginning. You can consume Serrano peppers and then work yourself to spicier pepper. Thai chilies are very spicy, so they have a maximum sirtuin-activating effect. But to get there, you have to take it easy. Slowly work yourself to the top. When buying these peppers, make sure you select the fresh ones with deep colors. You need to avoid the soft and wrinkled ones.

Cocoa

Cocoa was considered sacred by the Aztecs and Mayans, and it was a food type reserved only for the warriors or the elite. It was often used as a currency, as people were aware of its value. Although back then, it was mostly used as a drink, you don't have to dilute it with milk or water to reap the full benefits of it. The best way to consume cocoa is by eating dark chocolate (with at least 85 percent solid cocoa). However, this also depends on how the chocolate is made, as this product is usually treated with an alkalizing agent, which is known to lower the acidity of the chocolate and give a darker color. This substance is also known to reduce sirtuin-activating flavanols. In the United States, food treated with this agent is properly labeled, but this measure doesn't apply worldwide. Most countries don't have such legislation to force food processors to label their products "processed with alkali." If you see such a product, I would advise you to avoid it, as this substance will prevent you from reaping the benefits of high cocoa percentage.

Coffee

This is a drink enjoyed by most adults out there, and it is considered indispensable by most of them. We even believe that we can function without a cup of coffee to start within the morning. That's not true, but we can honestly believe that coffee significantly improves our productivity and our daily activities. The caffeine acid is a nutrient known to activate sirtuins, so there's more to drinking coffee than a popular and a very pleasant social activity. Coffee houses all over the world are making serious money out of people's addiction to hanging out and drinking coffee. It is no secret that coffee is very good for your metabolism. It boosts your energy level, so you can even work out at full intensity. However, you don't want to drink too much coffee, as coffee excess can be harmful to your blood pressure. Most specialists would agree that 2 to 4 cups of coffee per day is the optimum daily quota. Some too many people can't stand the taste of coffee and put a lot of sugar on it. Whether you use regular sugar, brown sugar, or even honey, I would rule them out. If you want to sweeten your coffee, use stevia instead or drink the coffee in its pure form.

Extra-Virgin Olive Oil

This oil is perhaps the healthiest form of fats you can think of, and it is not missing from any salad in the Mediterranean diet. The health benefits of consuming this oil are countless. It prevents and fights against diabetes, different types of cancer, osteoporosis, and many more. Plus, the extra-virgin olive oil can be associated with increased longevity, as it also has anti-aging effects. You can easily find this type of oil in most supermarkets, so you don't have any excuse to exclude it from your sirtfood diet. This oil has the right nutrients to activate the sirtuin gene in your body.

Garlic

I don't know about you guys, but I'm simply in love with garlic. I'm sure I'm not the only one. Forget about the smell it leaves behind. Enjoy the great taste it offers. I would have garlic with any meal. Of course, this may not fit with our busy lifestyle, as it is not recommended to have it before a meeting, but you can enjoy it for dinner or at home. But there's more to the consumption of garlic. As you probably know, it has an antifungal and antibiotic effect and has been successfully used to treat stomach ulcers. Plus, it can be used to remove waste products from your body. It has amazing effects on your blood pressure, blood sugar level, and your heart. So why refuse this delicious food to feel healthy? Garlic contains allicin, a nutrient capable of triggering sirtuins, but this nutrient can only be valued if the garlic clove is crushed. Therefore, if you want to reap the benefits of this food, you have to avoid cooking it immediately. You need to crush it first and let the allicin form (should take around 10 minutes) before cooking it. This is the right way to use garlic in a sirtfood diet.

Green Tea

In some cultures, drinking tea is as popular as drinking coffee, but what if you find the tea assortment that works best for you? You can indeed have tea from various medicinal plants, and they all have positive effects on your health. However, most of these plants are focused on preventing or fighting a specific disease. Have you ever thought about drinking tea for your well-being or to feel great? Well, this is what green tea is for. It first appeared in Asia, green tea has become very popular in Western culture. It has plenty of antioxidants. It can be used for detox, and it speeds up your metabolism. But there's a lot more to drinking green tea than these. Its benefits expand to preventing and fighting against diabetes, heart diseases, and cancer in developing forms. When it comes to sirtuins activation, green tea contains EGCG (epigallocatechin), which is known to be a very powerful sirtuin activator.

Well, this is what normal green tea can do for you, but if you want more obvious results, then you need to go for the matcha tea, which is the super green tea. This form of green tea is powdered, and it gets dissolved directly in the water, unlike normal green tea, which is prepared through an infusion. Therefore, this method of preparation allows the tea to have seriously increased levels of EGCG, in comparison with other forms of green tea. It is no wonder why Zen priests consider matcha as the ultimate medical and mental remedy.

CHAPTER 5
WHAT ARE THE STEPS TO APPLY THE DIET?

The Sirtfood Diet has two phases that last a total of three weeks. After that, you can continue "sirtifying" your diet by including as many sirtfoods as possible in your meals.

The specific recipes for these two phases are found in The Sirtfood Diet book, which was written by the diet's creators. You'll need to purchase it to follow the diet.

The meals are full of sirtfoods but do include other ingredients besides just the "top 20 sirtfoods."

Most of the ingredients and sirtfoods are easy to find.

However, three of the signature ingredients required for these two phases — matcha green tea powder, lovage and buckwheat — may be expensive or difficult to find.

A big part of the diet is its green juice, which you'll need to make yourself between one and three times daily. You will need a juicer (a blender will not work) and a kitchen scale, as the ingredients are listed by weight. The recipe is below:

Sirtfood Green Juice

- 75 grams (2.5 oz) kale

- 30 grams (1 oz) arugula (rocket)

- 5 grams parsley

- 2 celery sticks

- 1 cm (0.5 in) ginger

- half a green apple

- half a lemon

- half a teaspoon matcha green tea

Juice all ingredients except for the green tea powder and lemon together, and pour them into a glass. Juice the lemon by hand, then stir both the lemon juice and green tea powder into your juice.

Phase One

The first phase lasts seven days and involves calorie restriction and lots of green juice. It is intended to jump-start your weight loss and claimed to help you lose 7 pounds (3.2 kg) in seven days.

During the first three days of phase one, calorie intake is restricted to 1,000 calories. You drink three green juices per day plus one meal. Each day you can choose from recipes in the book, which all involve sirtfoods as a main part of the meal.

Meal examples include miso-glazed tofu, the sirtfood omelet or a shrimp stir-fry with buckwheat noodles.

On days 4–7 of phase one, calorie intake is increased to 1,500. This includes two green juices per day and two more sirtfood-rich meals, which you can choose from the book.

Phase Two

Phase two lasts for two weeks. During this "maintenance" phase, you should continue to steadily lose weight.

There is no specific calorie limit for this phase. Instead, you eat three meals full of sirtfoods and one green juice per day. Again, the meals are chosen from recipes provided in the book.

After the Diet

You may repeat these two phases as often as desired for further weight loss.

However, you are encouraged to continue "sirtifying" your diet after completing these phases by incorporating sirtfoods regularly into your meals.

There are a variety of Sirtfood Diet books that are full of recipes rich in sirtfoods. You can also include sirtfoods in your diet as a snack or in recipes you already use.

Additionally, you are encouraged to continue drinking the green juice every day.

In this way, the Sirtfood Diet becomes more of a lifestyle change than a one-time diet.

Eating some quality foods will improve your "skinny gene" pathways and enables you to shed some unnecessary weight in seven days. Food such as kale, dark chocolate, and wine has a natural compound known as polyphenols that look likes the results of fitness workout and fasting. Strawberries, cinnamon, as well as turmeric, are also strong sirtfoods. These foods will activate sirtuin steps or potential to help improve weight loss.

There are two stages to follow the sirtfood diet:

STAGE 1

through the first three days, calorie consumption is reduced to 1,000, which is more than on a 5:2 fasting day. The diet involves 3 Sirtfood-full of green juices and 1 Sirtfood filled meal, and 2 serves of dark chocolate.

For the residual four days, calorie intake has to be increased to 1, 500 calories, and the daily day the diet should involve 2 Sirtfood- filled green juices and 2 Sirtfood-rich meals.

In stage one, you are not permitted to drink any alcohol, but you are free to take water and green tea.

STAGE 2

Stage 2 does not center on calorie intake reduction. Daily intake involves 3 Sirtfood-rich foods and one green juice, and the alternative of 1 or 2 Sirtfood crunch snacks, if necessary.

In the second stage, you can take red wine, 2-3 glasses of red wine weekly at most, and also water, tea, coffee, and green tea.

You may replicate these two stages as much you desired for additional weight loss.

However, you are advised to continue "sirtifying" your diet at the end of completing these phases by including sirtfoods frequently into your meals.

There are differences in Sirtfood Diet manuals that have several recipes rich in sirtfoods. Also, you are advised to continue taking the green juice daily.

In this manner, the Sirtfood Diet will be more of a way of lifestyle adjustment than a one-time diet

It's no accident that some of the individuals with long lifespan and healthiest populations in the world eat diets that are rich in these sirtuin-activating foods; examples are those in the Mediterranean and parts of Asia. The Mediterranean diet includes polyphenol-rich fruits, veggies, olive oil, plus red wine. The Asian diet is rich in isoflavones present in soya beans and epigallactins from green Tea.

Acquiring several of these healthy foods into your diet is primary. They can be included in many diets and even compound to make super-sirt meals!

These are some ideas from which you can start:

Use olive oil for frying or roasting veggies or vegetables and salad dressings.

Include tofu or tempeh to stir-fries. Mix silken tofu into soups, immerse, and creamy desserts.

Put berries, blackcurrants to muesli, smoothies, and juices. Fresh yogurt, as well as fresh berries, ensure a healthy snack or dessert. Ensure to own a jar of olives handy to snack on and include olives to salads or cooked meals. Tapenade usually makes an excellent topping for rye bread.

Take your greens.

Cabbage and broccoli are outstanding support for any meal.

Curries, stews, and casseroles—exchange the usual Tea and coffee for green tea. Include a press of lemon for extra interest.

Miso alternatively can be used rather than stock cubes to flavor soups and stews. Milder light-colored miso may be used as a spread. Miso soup makes a great snack or soft meal if presented with salad or bread.

Apples are the ideal handy snack. Make sure you have one with you most times. Take your greens. Cabbage and broccoli are outstanding support to any meal and can also be included in stir-fries, curries, stews, and casseroles.

Enrich up your life with turmeric and other spices. Don't limit your input of seasonings to curries, include them to grains and vegetables.

Include cacao powder to smoothies and desserts too. Dredge cacao nibs on salads or include to trail mixes.

Buckwheat macaroni can be made as a tasty gluten complimentary option to wheat pasta, and buckwheat flour can also be made in baked products or to stiffer sauces. Buckwheat is also a great alternative that goes well with salads combined with roasted vegetables and toasted nuts.

The sirtfood diet is mainly followed in two different phases or steps. In the first step, a person needs to reduce his caloric intake to 1000 calories per day and take green juices three times a day along with sirtfood. After a week of this regime, the dieter can enter into the second phase in which he can focus more on the sirtfood and decrease the green juice intake down to once per day. These two phases can be repeated or continued for a longer duration to achieve a lasting weight loss goal.

Phase 1

The first 7-days of this diet plan are group together as Phase One. In this phase, the Sirt food dieter must rely on calorie restriction technique and continue consuming green juices. These seven days are essential to start your weight loss process, and usually, it is these days that help you lose weight up to 7 pounds the dieter follows the diet properly. If you find yourself successful at meeting this target, that means that you are doing great.

In its first three days, the dieter must reduce his caloric intake down to 1000 calories.

Besides restricting the caloric consumption, the dieter must also consume green juice throughout the day, about three times a day. It is suggested to drink green juice after or before every meal. The recipes given in this cookbook are perfect for selecting a variety of green juices of your choice. Moreover, there are several meal options available that can ensure low caloric intake; all you have to do is to pick the right meal from this cookbook. When the first three days of this diet passes, the dieter can increase the caloric intake up to 1500 calories a day. The next four days are also crucial, and the dieter must reduce the green juices to two times in a day. And take these juices along with more of the sirtfood.

Phase 2

The end of the first phase of the sirtfood diet marks phase two. This phase is all about the maintenance and regulation of the diet that you have initially started. As the first phase prepares the body to accept the dietary changes and work accordingly, the second phase is the result yielding stage, provided that the dieter follows it appropriately. This phase allows the body to continue working towards the weight loss goals steadily and progressively. That is the reason that the overall duration of the stage is nearly two weeks.

In this second phase, there is no such caloric restriction as it is in the case of the first phase. In this phase, as long as the dieter is consuming food that is rich in sirtuins for three times a day, it is considered appropriate to achieve all the weight loss goals, because by now the body is already tuned as a result of the first phase. Instead of consuming green juices about three -two times per day, the dieter can now drink one glass of juice a day, and that will be enough to maintain the accelerated rates of metabolism. When to take the juice depends on you, either to take the juice after the meal or before it.

CHAPTER 6
SIRTFOOD AROUND THE WORLD

Here are nine easy Sirtfood snacks you can reach for when you need a SIRT top-up.

1. Green tea

1 cup (200ml) • 1 of your SIRT 5 a day • 0 calories

Never, ever, underestimate the healthy SIRT boost that a cup of green tea can give you. Have as many cups as you can per day – we recommend at least two cups. Not only that, the SIRTs in green tea are cumulative so you can get up to four portions of SIRTs daily if you have four cups of green tea or more.

2. Red grapes

10 grapes • 1 of your SIRT 5 a day • 30 calories

Another of the very easy Sirtfood snacks and a low-calorie way to get one of your SIRT portions. Keep a punnet or two in the fridge and have a handful at breakfast or lunch or even both!

3. Apples

1 apple • 1 of your SIRT 5 a day • 47 calories

An apple a day really does keep the doctor away. Reach for an apple as one of your after-lunch easy Sirtfood snacks. It will help keep sugar cravings at bay too.

4. Cocoa

2 tsp/10g cocoa • 1 of your SIRT 5 a day • 33 calories

Try making a chocolate shot with 2 tsp cocoa. 1 tsp sugar and 30ml milk. Mix the cocoa and sugar together with a little boiling water from the kettle to make a smooth paste. Stir in the milk. An (almost) instant chocolate hit with only 68 calories.

5. Olives

6 large black or green olives • 1 of your SIRT 5 a day • 75 calories

A versatile and easy Sirtfood snack in the afternoon or a pre-dinner treat. Serve at room temperature to get a fuller flavor.

6. Blackberries

15 blackberries • 1 of your SIRT 5 a day • 32 calories

Another of the easy Sirtfood snacks to keep in your fridge. Also great as a frozen treat.

7. Dark chocolate 85%

6 squares/20g chocolate • 1 of your SIRT 5 a day • 125 calories

Get your chocolate hit here! If you prefer 70% dark chocolate, you'll need 9 squares/30g. which will be 180 calories.

8. Pomegranate seeds

50g/half a small pack • 1 of your SIRT 5 a day • 50 calories

Easy to obtain while on the go, pomegranate seeds pack a large SIRT punch and you only need half a 100g pack to get one of your SIRT portions.

9. Blueberries

25 blueberries (80g) • 1 of your sirt 5 a day • 36 cals

One large handful of blueberries can also be one of your easy Sirtfood snacks.

10. Honey Chilli Nuts

150g (5oz) walnuts □ 150g (5oz) pecan nuts □ 50g (2oz) softened butter □ 1 tablespoon honey

½ bird's-eye chilli, very finely chopped and de-seeded

Preheat the oven to 180C/360F. Combine the butter, honey and chilli in a bowl then add the nuts and stir them well. Spread the nuts onto a lined baking sheet and roast them in the oven for 10 minutes, stirring once halfway through. Remove from the oven and allow them to cool before eating.

Sirtfoods With Other Foods

We know that Sirtfoods and some other foods are good for us, whether its veggies like broccoli or tomatoes, spices like turmeric, or beverages like green tea. The reason these – and many other plant foods – are good for us, is primarily down to the bio-active plant compounds they contain. For the nutritionally savvy, we might be thinking of sulforaphane from broccoli, lycopene from tomatoes, curcumin from turmeric, and catechins from green tea. All the subject of extensive scientific research that goes a long way to explaining just why these foods are so good for our health.

But rather than just eating those individual foods, as good as they are, what if mixing certain foods – and therefore their nutrients – together at meals delivered an even bigger health boost? What if we could create synergies between nutrients in different foods that amplify their health benefits? It's a new idea, and here are a top-five of examples of how foods can add up for maximum effect.

1. Green tea + lemon: Green tea drinkers can expect numerous health benefits given that consuming this prized beverage is linked with less cancer, heart disease, diabetes and osteoporosis. These health benefits can be explained by its exceptional content of plant compounds called catechins, and especially a type called epigallocatechin gallate (EGCG). Adding a squeeze of lemon juice to your green tea, which is rich in vitamin C, helps to significantly increase the amount of catechins that get absorbed into the body.

2. Tomato sauce + extra virgin olive oil: Lycopene is the carotenoid responsible for the deep red color of tomatoes, and its consumption is linked with a reduced risk of certain cancers (most notably cancer of the prostate), cardiovascular disease, osteoporosis, and even protecting the skin from the damaging effects of the sun. The first thing to know about lycopene is that cooking and processing tomatoes dramatically increases the amount of lycopene that the body can absorb. The second is that the presence of fat further increases lycopene absorption. So teaming up your tomato-based dishes with a generous drizzle of extra virgin olive oil makes perfect sense.

3. Turmeric + black pepper: Turmeric, the bright yellow spice ever-present in traditional Indian cooking, is the subject of intense scientific study for its anti-cancer properties, it's potential to reduce inflammation in the body, and even for staving off dementia. This is believed to be primarily due to its active constituent curcumin. But the problem with curcumin is that it is very poorly absorbed by the body. However, adding black pepper increases its absorption, making them the perfect spice double-act. Cooking turmeric in liquid, and adding fat, further helps with curcumin absorption.

4. Broccoli + mustard: It's no secret that broccoli is good for us, with benefits including reducing cancer risk. Broccoli's main cancer-preventive ingredient is sulforaphane. This is formed when we eat broccoli by the action of an enzyme found in broccoli called myrosinase. However, cooking broccoli – especially over-cooking it – begins

to destroy the myrosinase enzyme, reducing the amount of sulforaphane that can be made. In fact, if we're not careful, we can cook the benefits right out of broccoli. However, for those who like their broccoli well-cooked (rather than lightly steamed for 2 to 4 minutes), adding in other natural sources of myrosinase, such as from mustard or horseradish, means that sulforaphane can still be made.

5. Salad + avocado: Green leafy vegetables such as kale, spinach and watercress, are packed full of health-promoting carotenoids such as immune-strengthening beta-carotene and eye-friendly lutein. However, when eaten raw, in the form of salads, these carotenoids are more difficult to absorb. But the addition of some fat can really help with that and adding avocado, rich in monounsaturated fat, to a salad, has been shown to dramatically increase the number of carotenoids that can be absorbed.

Enjoy the Sirtfoods with additions and reap the added health benefits.

CHAPTER 7
RECIPES
BREAKFAST

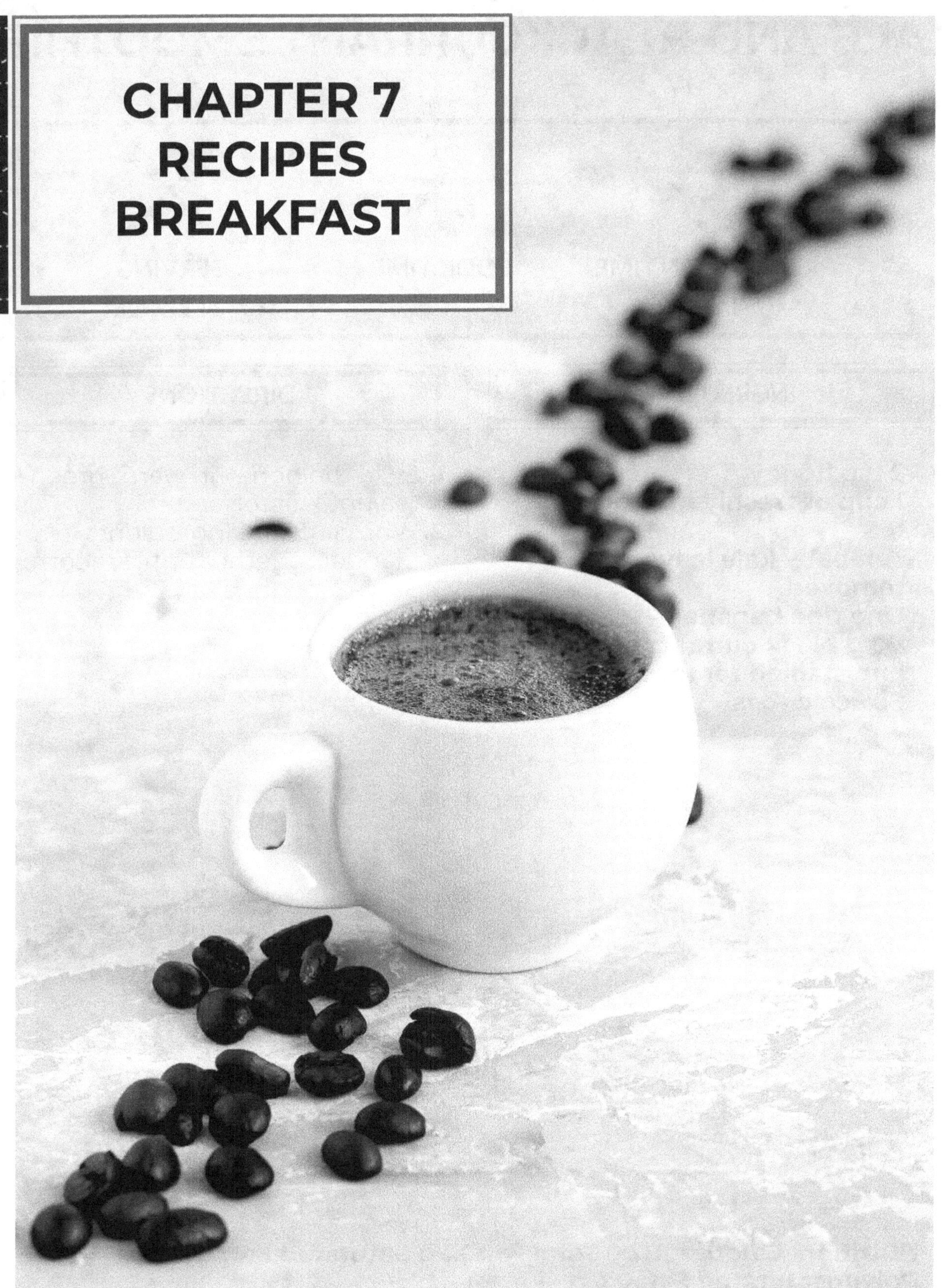

KALE AND BLACKCURRANT SMOOTHIE

PREPARATION TIME
3 MINUTES

COOK TIME
0

SERVING
2 PEOPLE

INGREDIENTS	DIRECTIONS

- **2 tsp honey**
- **1 cup of freshly made green tea**
- **Ten baby kale leaves stalk removed**
- **One ripe banana**
- **40 g black currants, washed and stalked removed**
- **Six ice cubes**

1. Swirl the honey in warm green tea until dissolved.
2. Whiz all of the ingredients in a blender together until smooth.
3. Serve straight away.

**Nutrition: Calories: 112.0 Total Fat: 1.1 g Saturated Fat: 0.2 g
Polyunsaturated Fat: 0.4 g
Monounsaturated Fat: 0.2 g Cholesterol: 0.0 mg Sodium: 16.3 mg
Potassium: 423.7 mg Total Carbohydrate: 26.9 g Dietary Fiber: 4.8 g
Sugars: 14.7 g Protein   2.1 g**

CHOCOLATE CUPCAKES WITH MATCHA ICING

PREPARATION TIME
12 MINUTES

COOK TIME
35 MINUTES

SERVING
2 PEOPLE

INGREDIENTS

- **150 g of self-reared flour,**
- **200 g of caster sugar,**
- **60 g of cocoa, 1/2 tsp of salt,**
- **1/2 tsp of excellent espresso coffee, decaf if desired,**
- **120ml of milk, 1/2 tsp of vanilla extract,**
- **50ml of vegetable oil,**
- **1 egg**
- **120ml of boiling water For the icing.**
- **50 g Butter, available at room temperature.**
- **50 g of icing sugar, 1 tbsp green tea powder**
- **1/2 tsp of vanilla bean paste, 50 g of cream soft cheese**

DIRECTIONS

1. Preheat the fan for the oven to 180C/160C. Fill a paper or silicone cake case with a cupcake tray.
2. In a large bowl, put the flour, sugar, cocoa, salt, and espresso powder and thoroughly mix in.
3. Pour in the boiling water carefully slowly and beat at low velocity until thoroughly combined. Use a fast beat to add air to the batter for another minute.
4. Gently spoon the batter between the cake cases. Each cake box should be no more than 3/4 complete. Bake 15-18 minutes in the oven until the mixture bounces back when squeezed. Extract from the oven and allow cooling before icing completely.
5. Mix the butter and sprinkle the sugar until it is light and smooth. Remove the coffee and Matcha powder, and stir again. Attach the cream cheese, then beat until smooth. Pip or brush over the cakes.

Nutrition:Calories: 302 Total Fat: 19g Saturated Fat: 10g Trans Fat: 0g Unsaturated Fat: 8g Cholesterol: 0mg Sodium: 129mg Carbohydrates: 31g Fiber: 3g Sugar: 16g Protein: 3g

GREEN TEA SMOOTHIE

PREPARATION TIME
3 MINUTES

COOK TIME
0

SERVING
2 PEOPLE

INGREDIENTS

- **2 ripe bananas**
- **250 ml milk**
- **2 tsp green tea powder Matcha**
- **1/2 tsp vanilla bean, or a small scrape of vanilla pod seeds**
- **Six ice cubes**
- **2 tsp honey**

DIRECTIONS

1. Easily combine all ingredients in a blender and serve in two glasses.

Nutrition: Calories: 282 Sugar: 37.6g Sodium: 56mg Fat: 6.1g Carbohydrates: 57.5g Fiber: 8.5g Protein: 5.6g

TURMERIC CHICKEN & KALE SALAD WITH HONEY-LIME

PREPARATION TIME
20 MINUTES

COOK TIME
10 MINUTES

SERVING
2 PEOPLE

INGREDIENTS

- **For the chicken**
- **One teaspoon ghee or 1 tbsp. coconut oil**
- **½ medium brown onion, diced**
- **250-300 g / 9 oz. chicken minces or diced up chicken thighs**
- **One large garlic clove, finely diced**
- **One teaspoon turmeric powder**
- **1teaspoon lime zest**
- **Juice of ½ limes**
- **½ salt + chili pepper**
- **For the salad**
- **Broccolini stalks 6 or 2 cups of broccoli florets**
- **Two tablespoons pumpkin seeds**
- **Large kale leaves 3, removed the stem and chopped**
- **½ Sliced Avocado**
- **A handful of fresh, chopped parsley leaves**

DIRECTIONS

1. Heat the ghee or coconut oil over medium-to-high heat in a small frying pan. Add the onion and sauté over medium heat for 4-5 minutes, until golden. Remove the slimy chicken and garlic, and swirl for 2-3 minutes over medium-high heat.
2. Add the turmeric, lime zest, salt, and pepper and cook, frequently stirring for another 3-4 minutes. Lay the cooked slush aside.
3. Bring a small water saucepan to boil while the chicken is cooking. Attach the broccolini, and cook for 2 minutes. Rinse under cold water, then break into 3 to 4 bits each.
4. Put the chicken pumpkin seeds into the frying pan and toast over medium heat for 2 minutes, frequently stirring to prevent burning. Also, use the fresh pumpkin seeds well.
5. Put the chopped kale in a salad bowl and pour over the dressing. Throw the kale with the oil, and rub it with the hands.
6. The cooked rice, broccolini, fresh herbs, pumpkin seeds, and slices of avocado are eventually tossed.

Nutrition: Calories 125 Calories: 551 Total Fat: 32g Saturated Fat: 5g Trans Fat: 0g Cholesterol: 70mg Sodium: 994mg Total Carbohydrate: 38g Dietary Fiber: 7g Sugars: 20g Protein: 36g

BAKED SALMON SALAD WITH CREAMY MINT

PREPARATION TIME
5 MINUTES

COOK TIME
20 MINUTES

SERVING
2 PEOPLE

INGREDIENTS

- **Ingredients:**
- **One salmon fillet (130g)**
- **40g mixed salad leaves**
- **40g young spinach leaves**
- **Two radishes, trimmed and thinly sliced**
- **5cm piece (50g) cucumber, cut into chunks**
- **Two spring onions, trimmed and sliced**
- **One small handful (10g) parsley, roughly chopped**
- **For the dressing:**
- **1 tsp low-fat mayonnaise**
- **1 tbsp natural yogurt**
- **1 tbsp. rice vinegar**
- **Two leave mint, finely chopped**
- **Salt and freshly ground black pepper**

DIRECTIONS

1. Preheat the oven to 200 ° C (fan/ gas 6 180 ° C).
2. Put the salmon filet on a baking tray and bake for 16–18 minutes until you have just cooked. Replace, and set aside from the oven. The salmon in the salad is equally lovely and hot or cold. If your salmon has skin, just cook the skin side down and remove the salmon from the skin after frying, using a slice of bread. When cooked, it should slide away quickly.
3. Mix the mayonnaise, yogurt, rice wine vinegar, mint leaves, and salt and pepper in a small bowl and let stand to allow the aromas to expand for at least 5 minutes.
4. Arrange on a serving plate, the salad leaves, and spinach, and top with the radishes, the cucumber, the spring onions, and the parsley. Flake the cooked salmon over the salad and brush over the dressing.

Nutrition: Calories: 282 Sugar: 37.6g Sodium: 56mg Fat: 6.1g Carbohydrates: 57.5g Fiber: 8.5g Protein: 5.6g

MAINS

COQ AU VIN

PREPARATION TIME
10 MINUTES

COOK TIME
40 MINUTES

SERVING
3 PEOPLE

INGREDIENTS

- **450g (1lb) button mushrooms**
- **100g (3½oz) streaky bacon, chopped**
- **16 chicken thighs, skin removed**
- **3 cloves of garlic, crushed**
- **3 tbsp fresh parsley, chopped**
- **3 carrots, chopped**
- **2 red onions, chopped**
- **2 tbsp plain flour**
- **2 tbsp olive oil**
- **750ml (1¼ pints) red wine**
- **1 bouquet garni**

DIRECTIONS

1. Place the flour on a large plate and coat the chicken in it.
2. Heat the olive oil in a large saucepan, add the chicken and brown it, before setting aside.
3. Fry the bacon in the pan, then add the onion and cook for 5 minutes.
4. Pour in the red wine and add the chicken, carrots, bouquet garni, and garlic.
5. Transfer it to a large ovenproof dish.
6. Cook in the oven at 180C/360F for 1 hour.
7. Remove the bouquet garni and skim off any excess fat, if necessary.
8. Add in the mushrooms and cook for 15 minutes.
9. Stir in the parsley just before serving.

Nutrition: Calories: 267.0 Total Fat: 8.7 g Saturated Fat: 1.8 g Polyunsaturated Fat: 1.1 g Monounsaturated Fat: 5.0 g Cholesterol: 77.6 mg Sodium : 145.7 mg Potassium: 525.5 mg Total Carbohydrate: 7.6 g Dietary Fiber: 1.0 g Sugars: 0.7 g Protein: 31.2 g

KALE WHITE BEAN PORK SOUP

 **PREPARATION TIME**
5 MINUTES

 **COOK TIME**
45 MINUTES

 **SERVING**
4-6 PEOPLE

INGREDIENTS

- **3 tbsp extra-virgin olive oil**
- **3 tbsp chili powder**
- **1 tbsp jalapeno hot sauce**
- **2 pounds bone-in pork chops**
- **Salt**
- **4 stalks celery, chopped**
- **1 large white onion, chopped**
- **3 cloves garlic, chopped**
- **2 cups chicken broth**
- **2 cups diced tomatoes**
- **2 cups cooked white beans**
- **6 cups packed kale**

DIRECTIONS

1. Preheat the broiler.
2. Whisk hot sauce, 1 tbsp olive oil, and chili powder in a bowl.
3. Season the pork chops with ½ tsp salt.
4. Rub chops with the spice mixture on both sides and place them on a rack set over a baking sheet.
5. Set aside.
6. Heat 1 tbsp olive oil in a pot over medium heat.
7. Add the celery, garlic, onion and the remaining 2 tbsp chili powder.
8. Cook until onions are translucent, stirring (approx. 8 minutes).
9. Add tomatoes and the chicken broth to the pot. Cook and occasionally stir until reduced by about one-third (approx. 7 minutes).
10. Add the kale and the beans.
11. Reduce the heat to medium, cover, and cook until the kale is tender (approx. 7 minutes).
12. Add up to ½ cup of water if the mixture looks dry and season with salt.
13. In the meantime, boil the pork until browned (approx. 4 to 6 minutes).
14. Flip and broil until cooked through.
15. Serve with the kale and beans.

Nutrition: Carbohydrates: 14 g Dietary Fiber: 3 g Sugar: 2 g Fat: 6 g Saturated: 2 g Protein: 7g

TURKEY SATAY SKEWERS

PREPARATION TIME	COOK TIME	SERVING
5 MINUTES	30 MINUTES	3 PEOPLE

INGREDIENTS

- **250g (9oz) turkey breast, cubed**
- **25g (1oz) smooth peanut butter**
- **1 clove of garlic, crushed**
- **½ small bird's eye chili (or more if you like it hotter), finely chopped**
- **½ tsp ground turmeric**
- **200ml (7fl oz) coconut milk**
- **2 tsp soy sauce**

DIRECTIONS

1. Combine the coconut milk, peanut butter, turmeric, soy sauce, garlic, and chili.
2. Add the turkey pieces to the bowl and stir them until they are completely coated.
3. Push the turkey onto metal skewers.
4. Place the satay skewers on a barbeque or under a hot grill (broiler) and cook for 4-5 minutes on each side, until they are completely cooked.

Nutrition: Carbohydrates: 6 g Dietary Fiber: 1 g Sugar: 2 g Fat: 12 g Saturated: 3 g Polyunsaturated: 3 g Monounsaturated: 5 g Trans: 0 g Protein: 66 g

TOMATO & GOAT'S CHEESE PIZZA

 **PREPARATION TIME**
5 MINUTES

 **COOK TIME**
40 MINUTES

 **SERVING**
3 PEOPLE

INGREDIENTS

- **225g (8oz) buckwheat flour**
- **2 tsp dried yeast**
- **Pinch of salt**
- **150ml (5fl oz) slightly water**
- **1 tsp olive oil**
- **For the topping:**
- **75g (3oz) feta cheese, crumbled**
- **75g (3oz) passata (or tomato paste)**
- **1 tomato, sliced**
- **1 red onion, finely chopped**
- **25g (1oz) rocket (arugula) leaves, chopped**

DIRECTIONS

1. In a bowl, combine all the ingredients for the pizza dough then allow it to stand for at least an hour until it has doubled in size.
2. Roll the dough out to a size to suit you.
3. Spoon the passata onto the base and add the rest of the toppings.
4. Bake in the oven at 200C/400F for 15-20 minutes or until browned at the edges and crispy and serve.

Nutrition: Calories 480. Calories from Fat 220. Total Fat 24g (37%) Saturated Fat 7g (35%) Cholesterol 25mg (8%) Sodium 770mg (32%) Total Carbohydrate 53g (18%) Dietary Fiber 3g (12%) Protein 14g. Vitamin A 10% Calcium 20% Iron 15%

TOFU THAI CURRY

PREPARATION TIME
5 MINUTES

COOK TIME
30 MINUTES

SERVING
3 PEOPLE

INGREDIENTS

- **400g (14oz) tofu, diced**
- **200g (7oz) sugar snap peas**
- **5cm (2-inch) chunk fresh ginger root, peeled and finely chopped**
- **2 red onions, chopped**
- **2 cloves of garlic, crushed**
- **2 bird's eye chilies**
- **2 tbsp tomato puree**
- **1 stalk of lemongrass, inner stalks only**
- **1 tbsp fresh coriander (cilantro), chopped**
- **1 tsp cumin**
- **300ml (½ pint) coconut milk**
- **200ml (7fl oz) vegetable stock (broth)**
- **1 tbsp virgin olive oil**
- **juice of 1 lime**

DIRECTIONS

1. Heat the oil in a frying pan, add the onion and cook for 4 minutes.
2. Add in the chilies, cumin, ginger, and garlic and cook for 2 minutes.
3. Add the tomato puree, lemongrass, sugar-snap peas, lime juice, and tofu and cook for 2 minutes.
4. Pour in the stock (broth), coconut milk and coriander (cilantro) and simmer for 5 minutes.
5. Serve with brown rice or buckwheat, and a handful of rocket (arugula) leaves on the side.

Nutrition: Carbohydrates: 6 g Dietary Fiber: 1 g Sugar: 2 g Fat: 12 g Saturated: 3 g Polyunsaturated: 3 g Monounsaturated: 5 g Trans: 0 g Protein: 66 g

TOMATO & GOAT'S CHEESE PIZZA

PREPARATION TIME
5 MINUTES

COOK TIME
40 MINUTES

SERVING
3 PEOPLE

INGREDIENTS

- **225g (8oz) buckwheat flour**
- **2 tsp dried yeast**
- **Pinch of salt**
- **150ml (5fl oz) slightly water**
- **1 tsp olive oil**
- **For the topping:**
- **75g (3oz) feta cheese, crumbled**
- **75g (3oz) passata (or tomato paste)**
- **1 tomato, sliced**
- **1 red onion, finely chopped**
- **25g (1oz) rocket (arugula) leaves, chopped**

DIRECTIONS

1. In a bowl, combine all the ingredients for the pizza dough then allow it to stand for at least an hour until it has doubled in size.
2. Roll the dough out to a size to suit you.
3. Spoon the passata onto the base and add the rest of the toppings.
4. Bake in the oven at 200C/400F for 15-20 minutes or until browned at the edges and crispy and serve.

Nutrition: Calories: 346.3 Total Fat: 26.4 g Saturated Fat: 2.0 g Polyunsaturated Fat: 5.7 g Monounsaturated Fat: 5.4 g Cholesterol: 0.0 mg Sodium: 364.4 mg Potassium: 356.9 mg Total Carbohydrate: 13.2 g Dietary Fiber: 3.1 g Sugars: 0.1 g Protein: 19.1 g

KALE WALNUT BAKE

PREPARATION TIME
10 MINUTES

COOK TIME
30 MINUTES

SERVING
4 PEOPLE

INGREDIENTS

- **1 medium red onion, finely chopped**
- **¼ cup extra virgin olive oil**
- **2 cups baby kale**
- **½ cup half-and-half cream**
- **½ cup walnuts, coarsely chopped**
- **1/3 cup dry breadcrumbs**
- **½ teaspoon ground nutmeg**
- **Salt and pepper to taste**
- **TOPPING:**
- **¼ cup dry breadcrumbs**
- **2 tablespoons extra virgin olive oil**

DIRECTIONS

1. Preheat oven to 350 degrees F.
2. In a skillet, sauté onion in olive oil until tender.
3. In a large bowl, combine cooked onion, kale, cream, walnuts, breadcrumbs, nutmeg, and salt and pepper to taste, mixing well.
4. Transfer to a greased 1-1/2-qt. Baking dish.
5. Combine topping ingredients and sprinkle over the kale mixture.
6. Bake, uncovered, for 30 minutes or until lightly browned.

Nutrition: Calories: 344.0 Total Fat: 29.0 g Saturated Fat: 5.8 g Polyunsaturated Fat: 6.3 g Monounsaturated Fat: 14.1 g Cholesterol: 10.7 mg Sodium : 560.4 mg Potassium: 632.5 mg Total Carbohydrate: 15.9 g Dietary Fiber: 5.8 g Sugars: 3.5 g Protein: 9.0 g

KALE-GREEN BEAN CASSEROLE

PREPARATION TIME	COOK TIME	SERVING
5 MINUTES	40 MINUTES	4 PEOPLE

INGREDIENTS

- 1 ½ cups milk
- 1 cup sour cream
- 1 cup mushrooms, chopped
- 2 cups green beans, chopped
- 2 cups kale, chopped
- ¼ cup capers, drained
- ¼ cup walnuts, crushed

DIRECTIONS

1. Preheat the oven to 375 degrees F and lightly grease a casserole dish.
2. Whisk the milk and sour cream together in a large bowl. Fold in the mushrooms, green beans, kale, and capers. Pour into the casserole dish and top with the crushed walnuts.
3. Bake uncovered in the preheated oven until bubbly and browned on top, about 40 minutes.

Nutrition: Calories: 138 calorie Total Fat: 8 grams Saturated Fat: 2 grams Cholesterol: 1 milligram Sodium: 830 milligrams Carbohydrates: 15 grams Dietary Fiber: 4 grams Protein: 5 grams Sugar: 5 grams

RICE WITH LEMON AND ARUGULA

PREPARATION TIME
10 MINUTES

COOK TIME
35 MINUTES

SERVING
4 PEOPLE

INGREDIENTS

- **1 small red onion, chopped**
- **1 cup fresh mushrooms, sliced**
- **2 cloves garlic, minced**
- **1 tablespoon extra virgin olive oil**
- **3 cups cooked long-grain rice**
- **1 (10 ounces) package fresh arugula**
- **3 tablespoons lemon juice**
- **¼ teaspoon dill weed**
- **Salt and pepper to taste**
- **1/3 cup feta cheese, crumbled**

DIRECTIONS

1. Preheat an oven to 350 degrees F
2. In a skillet, sauté the onion, mushrooms, and garlic in oil until tender. Stir in the rice, arugula, lemon juice, dill and salt and pepper to taste.
3. Reserve 1 tablespoon cheese and stir the rest into skillet; mix well.
4. Transfer to an 8-in. Square baking dish coated with nonstick cooking spray. Sprinkle with reserved cheese.
5. Cover and bake for 25 minutes.
6. Uncover and bake for an additional 5-10 minutes or until heated through, and cheese is melted.

Nutrition: Calories: 164.3 Total Fat: 15.6 g Saturated Fat: 3.0 g Polyunsaturated Fat: 1.3 g Monounsaturated Fat: 10.5 g Cholesterol: 4.8 mg Sodium: 195.7 mg Potassium: 124.3 mg Total Carbohydrate: 5.7 g Dietary Fiber: 2.1 g Sugars: 0.3 g Protein: 3.5 g

CAJUN TURKEY STUFFING

PREPARATION TIME
10 MINUTES

COOK TIME
25 MINUTES

SERVING
6-8 PEOPLE

INGREDIENTS

- **5 quarts chicken broth**
- **10 cups uncooked white rice**
- **1 ½ cups celery, chopped**
- **1 ½ cups red onion, chopped**
- **1 tablespoon garlic, minced**
- **1 pound ground pork**
- **1 pound ground beef**
- **2 tablespoons Cajun seasoning**
- **1 tablespoon dried thyme**
- **1 tablespoon dried parsley**
- **1 tablespoon dried oregano**

DIRECTIONS

1. Place the chicken broth, rice, celery, and 1 cup of chopped onion into a large pot. Bring to a boil over high heat.
2. Reduce heat to medium-low, cover, and simmer until the rice is tender, 20 to 25 minutes.
3. Meanwhile, place the remaining ½ cup of onion into a large skillet along with the garlic, pork, and beef. Cook and stir over medium-high heat until the meat is brown and crumbly.
4. Pour off excess grease, then stir the meat into the cooked rice along with the thyme, parsley, and oregano. Stir well.

Nutrition: Calories: 445 Total fat: 8.3 g Cholesterol: 27 mg Sodium: 228 mg 76 g carbohydrates Protein: 13.8 g

PURPLE POTATOES WITH ONIONS, MUSHROOMS, AND CAPERS

PREPARATION TIME
10 MINUTES

COOK TIME
25 MINUTES

SERVING
4 PEOPLE

INGREDIENTS

- **6 purple potatoes, scrubbed**
- **3 tablespoons extra virgin olive oil**
- **1 large red onion, chopped**
- **8 ounces fresh mushrooms, sliced**
- **Salt and pepper to taste**
- **¼ teaspoon chili pepper flakes**
- **1 tablespoon capers, drained and chopped**
- **1 teaspoon fresh tarragon, chopped**

DIRECTIONS

1. Cut each potato into wedges by quartering the potatoes, then cutting each quarter in half.
2. Heat 1 tablespoon of olive oil over medium heat in a large skillet and cook the onion and mushrooms until the mushrooms start to release their liquid. The onion becomes translucent for about 5 minutes. Transfer the onion and mushrooms into a bowl and set aside.
3. Heat 2 more tablespoons of olive oil over high heat in the same skillet and add the potato wedges into the hot oil. Sprinkle with salt and pepper, and allow to cook, occasionally stirring, until the wedges are browned on both sides, about 10 minutes.
4. Reduce heat to medium, sprinkle the potato wedges with red pepper flakes, and allow to cook until the potatoes are tender about 10 more minutes. Stir in the onion and mushroom mixture, toss the vegetables together, and mix in the capers and fresh tarragon.

Nutrition:Calories:188.6 Protein: 4.5 g Carbohydrates: 29.7 g Cholesterol: 0 mg Sodium: 45.5 mg

CAJUN TURKEY STUFFING

PREPARATION TIME
10 MINUTES

COOK TIME
25 MINUTES

SERVING
6-8 PEOPLE

INGREDIENTS

- **5 quarts chicken broth**
- **10 cups uncooked white rice**
- **1 ½ cups celery, chopped**
- **1 ½ cups red onion, chopped**
- **1 tablespoon garlic, minced**
- **1 pound ground pork**
- **1 pound ground beef**
- **2 tablespoons Cajun seasoning**
- **1 tablespoon dried thyme**
- **1 tablespoon dried parsley**
- **1 tablespoon dried oregano**

DIRECTIONS

1. Place the chicken broth, rice, celery, and 1 cup of chopped onion into a large pot. Bring to a boil over high heat.
2. Reduce heat to medium-low, cover, and simmer until the rice is tender, 20 to 25 minutes.
3. Meanwhile, place the remaining ½ cup of onion into a large skillet along with the garlic, pork, and beef. Cook and stir over medium-high heat until the meat is brown and crumbly.
4. Pour off excess grease, then stir the meat into the cooked rice along with the thyme, parsley, and oregano. Stir well.

Nutrition: Calories: 445 Total fat: 8.3 g Cholesterol: 27 mg Sodium: 228 mg 76 g carbohydrates Protein: 13.8 g

KING PRAWN STIR-FRY WITH BUCKWHEAT NOODLES

PREPARATION TIME
5 MINUTES

COOK TIME
40 MINUTES

SERVING
2 PEOPLE

INGREDIENTS

- **75g of soba buckwheat noodles**
- **1 bird's eye chili, finely chopped**
- **5g of lovage or celery leaves**
- **2 teaspoons of extra virgin olive oil**
- **20g of red onions, sliced**
- **75g of green beans, chopped**
- **50g of kale, roughly chopped**
- **100ml chicken stock**
- **40g of celery, trimmed and sliced**
- **2 teaspoons of tamari**
- **1 teaspoon of finely chopped fresh ginger**
- **150g of shelled raw king prawns, deveined**
- **1 garlic clove, finely chopped**

DIRECTIONS

1. Place a frying pan over high heat and add a teaspoon of tamari and oil.
2. Cook the prawns in the oil for 2 to 3 minutes then place them on a plate.
3. Place the noodles in boiling water and cook for 5 to 8 minutes. Drain, and then set aside.
4. Use the remaining oil to fry the garlic, beans, red onion, chili, ginger, celery, and kale in a pan for 2 to 3 minutes over medium-high heat. Add the stock, let it boil, and then simmer for 2 minutes, or until the vegetables are crunchy cooked.
5. Add the celery/lovage, prawns, and noodles to the pan and let it boil. Remove from heat and serve.

Nutrition: Total Fat: 11.2 g Cholesterol: 63mg Sodium: 1909mg Carbohydrates: 70g Protein: 43g

PRAWN & CHILI PAK CHOI

 **PREPARATION TIME**
5 MINUTES

 **COOK TIME**
35 MINUTES

 **SERVING**
4 PEOPLE

INGREDIENTS

- **75g brown rice**
- **1 pak choi**
- **60ml chicken stock**
- **1 tbsp extra virgin olive oil**
- **1 garlic clove, finely chopped**
- **50g red onion, finely chopped**
- **½ bird's eye chili, finely chopped**
- **1 tsp freshly grated ginger**
- **125g shelled raw king prawns**
- **1 tbsp soy sauce**
- **1 tsp five-spice**
- **1 tbsp freshly chopped flat-leaf parsley**
- **A pinch of salt and pepper**

DIRECTIONS

1. Place a frying pan over high heat and add a teaspoon of tamari and oil.
2. Cook the prawns in the oil for 2 to 3 minutes then place them on a plate.
3. Place the noodles in boiling water and cook for 5 to 8 minutes. Drain, and then set aside.
4. Use the remaining oil to fry the garlic, beans, red onion, chili, ginger, celery, and kale in a pan for 2 to 3 minutes over medium-high heat. Add the stock, let it boil, and then simmer for 2 minutes, or until the vegetables are crunchy cooked.
5. Add the celery/lovage, prawns, and noodles to the pan and let it boil. Remove from heat and serve.

Nutrition: Total Fat: 11.2 g Cholesterol: 63mg Sodium: 1909mg Carbohydrates: 70g Protein: 43g

PRAWN & CHILI PAK CHOI

PREPARATION TIME	COOK TIME	SERVING
5 MINUTES	35 MINUTES	4 PEOPLE

INGREDIENTS

- **75g brown rice**
- **1 pak choi**
- **60ml chicken stock**
- **1 tbsp extra virgin olive oil**
- **1 garlic clove, finely chopped**
- **50g red onion, finely chopped**
- **½ bird's eye chili, finely chopped**
- **1 tsp freshly grated ginger**
- **125g shelled raw king prawns**
- **1 tbsp soy sauce**
- **1 tsp five-spice**
- **1 tbsp freshly chopped flat-leaf parsley**
- **A pinch of salt and pepper**

DIRECTIONS

1. Bring a medium-sized saucepan of water to the boil and cook the brown rice for 25-30 minutes, or until softened.
2. Tear the pak choi into pieces. Warm the chicken stock in a skillet over medium heat and toss in the pak choi, cooking until the pak choi has slightly wilted.
3. In another skillet, warm olive oil over high heat. Toss in the ginger, chili, red onions and garlic frying for 2-3 minutes.
4. Throw in the pawns, five-spice and soy sauce and cook for 6-8 minutes, or until the cooked throughout. Drain the brown rice and add to the skillet, stirring and cooking for 2-3 minutes. Add the pak choi, garnish with parsley and serve.

Nutrition: Cabohydrates: 8.8g Fiber: 4.0g Protein: 15.9g Fat: 6.3g
Saturates: 0.50g Sugars: 7.0g Salt: 0.90g

SMOKED SALMON OMELET

PREPARATION TIME
5 MINUTES

COOK TIME
45 MINUTES

SERVING
1 PEOPLE

INGREDIENTS

- **10g of chopped Rocket**
- **100g smoked salmon, sliced**
- **1 teaspoon of extra virgin olive oil**
- **½ teaspoon of capers**
- **2 medium eggs**
- **1 teaspoon of chopped Parsley**

DIRECTIONS

1. Crack the eggs into a bowl and whisk them well. Add the capers, parsley, rocket, and salmon and heat oil in a non-stick pan until hot but not smoking.
2. Add the egg mixture into the pan and move it around the pan using a spatula.
3. Reduce the heat to low and let the omelet cook. Slide the spatula under the omelet, fold it up in half, and serve.

Nutrition: Calories: 288.1 Total Fat: 9.2 g Saturated Fat: 2.4 g Polyunsaturated Fat: 1.8 g Monounsaturated Fat: 3.5 g Cholesterol: 205.6 mg Sodium   2: 112.5 mg Potassium: 318.9 mg Total Carbohydrate: 15.6 g Dietary Fiber: 3.1 g Sugars: 0.8 g Protein: 33.1 g

MUSSELS IN RED WINE SAUCE

PREPARATION TIME
5 MINUTES

COOK TIME
50 MINUTES

SERVING
2 PEOPLE

INGREDIENTS

- **800g 2lb mussels**
- **2 x 400g 14 oz tins of chopped tomatoes**
- **25g 1oz butter**
- **1 tablespoon fresh chives, chopped**
- **1 tablespoon fresh parsley, chopped**
- **1 bird's-eye chili, finely chopped**
- **4 cloves of garlic, crushed**
- **400 ml 14fl. oz red wine**
- **Juice of 1 lemon**

DIRECTIONS

1. Wash the mussels, remove their beards, and set them aside.
2. Heat the butter in a large saucepan and add in the red wine.
3. Reduce the heat and add the parsley, chives, chili, and garlic while stirring.
4. Add in the tomatoes, lemon juice, and mussels.
5. Cover the saucepan and cook for 2-3 minutes.
6. Remove the saucepan from the heat and take out any mussels which haven't opened and discard them.
7. Serve and eat immediately.

Nutrition: Calories: 388.9 Total Fat: 15.2 g Saturated Fat: 4.3 g Polyunsaturated Fat: 2.4 g Monounsaturated Fat: 5.9 g Cholesterol: 94.8 mg Sodium : 617.9 mg Potassium: 595.3 mg Total Carbohydrate: 18.0 g Dietary Fiber: 0.4 g Sugars: 0.6 g Protein: 37.2 g

GINGER PRAWN STIR-FRY

PREPARATION TIME
5 MINUTES

COOK TIME
50 MINUTES

SERVING
1 PEOPLE

INGREDIENTS

- **6 prawns or shrimp peeled and deveined**
- **½ package of buckwheat noodles called Soba in Asian sections**
- **5-6 leaves of kale, chopped**
- **1 cup of green beans, chopped**
- **5 g lovage or celery leaves**
- **1 garlic clove, finely chopped**
- **1 bird's eye chili, finely chopped**
- **1 tsp fresh ginger, finely chopped**
- **2 stalks celery, chopped**
- **½ small red onion, chopped**
- **1 cup chicken stock or vegetable if you prefer**
- **2 tbsp. soy sauce**
- **2 tbsp. extra virgin olive oil**

DIRECTIONS

1. Cook prawns in a bit of the oil and soy sauce until done and set aside about 10-15 minutes).
2. Boil the noodles according to the Directions usually 6-8 minutes). Set aside.
3. Sauté the vegetables, then add the garlic, ginger, red onion, chili in a bit of oil until tender and crunchy, but not mushy. Add the prawns, and noodles, and simmer low about 5-10 minutes past that point.

Nutrition: Calories: 92.0 Total Fat: 2.2 g Saturated Fat: 0.2 g Polyunsaturated Fat: 0.1 g Monounsaturated Fat: 0.8 g Cholesterol: 113.3 mg Sodium: 430.3 mg Potassium: 47.2 mg Total Carbohydrate: 3.2 g Dietary Fiber: 0.2 g Sugars: 0.0 g Protein:14.7 g

TURKEY MOLE TACOS

PREPARATION TIME
5 MINUTES

COOK TIME
25 MINUTES

SERVING
3 PEOPLE

INGREDIENTS

- **Lean ground turkey - .75 pound**
- **Green onion, chopped – 4 stalks**
- **Garlic cloves, minced – 2**
- **Celery, chopped – 1 rib**
- **Roasted sweet peppers, chopped and drained – 3.5 ounces**
- **Diced tomatoes, canned – 7 ounces**
- **Corn tortillas, 6 inches, warmed – 6**
- **Red onion, thinly sliced – 1**
- **Walnuts, roasted, chopped – 2 tablespoons**
- **Dark chocolate, chopped – 2 ounces**
- **Sea salt - .25 teaspoon**
- **Chili powder – 4 teaspoons**
- **Cumin - .5 teaspoon**
- **Cinnamon, ground - .125 teaspoon**

DIRECTIONS

1. In a large non-stick skillet, cook the ground turkey with the green onions, celery, and garlic over medium heat. Cook until there is no pink remaining, the turkey has reached a temperature of one-hundred and sixty-five degrees, and the vegetables are tender.
2. Into the skillet with the cooked turkey, add the canned tomatoes, roasted red peppers, cinnamon, chocolate, chili powder, cumin, and sea salt. Allow the liquid from the tomatoes to come to a boil before reducing the heat to medium-low, cover the skillet with a lid, and simmer for ten minutes. Stir occasionally to prevent sticking and burning.
3. Remove the cooked ground turkey from the heat and stir in the walnuts.
4. Divide the taco meat between the corn tortillas, topping it off with the sliced red onion. Serve while warm.

Nutrition:Calories: 369 Fat 15g (5g saturated fat) Cholesterol: 75mg Sodium: 612mg, Carbohydrate: 37g(8g sugars, 6g fiber) Protein: 22g

CHICKEN WITH BALSAMIC ONIONS AND MUSHROOMS

PREPARATION TIME
5 MINUTES

COOK TIME
40 MINUTES

SERVING
6 PEOPLE

INGREDIENTS

- **Chicken thighs, boneless and skinless – 3**
- **Sea salt – .5 teaspoon**
- **Chicken broth - .25 cup**
- **Mushrooms, sliced – 4 ounces**
- **Extra virgin olive oil – 1.5 tablespoons, divided**
- **Onion, thinly sliced – 1**
- **Heavy cream – .5 tablespoon**
- **Balsamic vinegar – 1 tablespoon**
- **Black pepper, ground - .25 teaspoon**

DIRECTIONS

1. Add one tablespoon of the extra virgin olive oil to a large skillet and sear the chicken thighs on each side over medium-high heat for four minutes. Remove the cooked chicken thighs from the large skillet and set it aside.
2. Into the skillet, add the remaining olive oil with the onions and saute them over medium-low heat until they caramelize, about fifteen minutes.
3. Stir the mushrooms into the skillet, cooking for five minute minutes until browned. Mix in the chicken broth, balsamic vinegar, and heavy cream. Nestle the chicken thighs into the mixture and continue to cook over medium heat until the chicken is cooked all the way through, about ten more minutes. The chicken is done when the internal temperature reaches Fahrenheit one-hundred and sixty-five degrees.

Nutrition: Calories: 190.9 Total Fat: 6.8 g Saturated Fat: 1.4 g Polyunsaturated Fat: 1.2 g Monounsaturated Fat: 3.5 g Cholesterol: 73.1 mg Sodium   : 264.7 mg Potassium: 270.8 mg Total Carbohydrate: 2.9 g Dietary Fiber: 0.6 g Sugars: 0.0 g Protein: 27.9 g

CHICKEN & BEAN CASSEROLE

PREPARATION TIME
5 MINUTES

COOK TIME
40 MINUTES

SERVING
2 PEOPLE

INGREDIENTS

- **400g 14ozchopped tomatoes**
- **400g 14 oz tinned cannellini beans or haricot beans**
- **8 chicken thighs, skin removed**
- **2 carrots, peeled and finely chopped**
- **2 red onions, chopped**
- **4 sticks of celery**
- **4 large mushrooms**
- **2 red peppers bell peppers, deseeded and chopped**
- **1 clove of garlic**
- **2 tablespoons soy sauce**
- **1 tablespoon olive oil**
- **1.75 liters 3 pints chicken stock broth**
- **509 calories per serving**

DIRECTIONS

1. Heat the olive oil in a saucepan, add the garlic and onions and cook for 5 minutes.
2. Add in the chicken and cook for 5 minutes, then add the carrots, cannellini beans, celery, red peppers bell peppers, and mushrooms.
3. Po reduce the heat and simmer for 45 minutes.
4. Serve with rice or new potatoes.

Nutrition: Bring it to the boil, Calories: 209.1 Total Fat: 6.6 g Saturated Fat: 2.5 g Polyunsaturated Fat: 0.4 g Monounsaturated Fat: 0.7 g Cholesterol: 79.3 mg Sodium: 667.9 mg Potassium: 306.9 mg Total Carbohydrate: 6.2 g Dietary Fiber: 3.2 g Sugars: 0.5 g Protein:31.0 g

CHICKEN CURRY WITH POTATOES AND KALE

PREPARATION TIME
10 MINUTES

COOK TIME
20 MINUTES

SERVING
4 PEOPLE

INGREDIENTS

- **600g chicken breast, cut into pieces**
- **4 tablespoons of extra virgin olive oil**
- **3 tablespoons turmeric**
- **2 red onions, sliced**
- **2 red chilies, finely chopped**
- **3 cloves of garlic, finely chopped**
- **1 tablespoon freshly chopped ginger**
- **1 tablespoon curry powder**
- **1 tin of small tomatoes (400ml)**
- **500ml chicken broth**
- **200ml coconut milk**
- **2 pieces cardamom**
- **1 cinnamon stick**
- **600g potatoes mainly waxy)**
- **10g parsley, chopped**
- **175g kale, chopped**
- **5g coriander, chopped**

DIRECTIONS

1. Marinate the chicken in a teaspoon of olive oil and a tablespoon of turmeric for about 30 minutes. Then fry in a high frying pan at high heat for about 4 minutes. Remove from the pan and set aside.
2. Heat a tablespoon of oil in a pan with chili, garlic, onion, and ginger. Boil everything over medium heat and then add the curry powder and a tablespoon of turmeric and cook for another two minutes, stirring occasionally. Add tomatoes, cook for another two minutes until finally chicken stock, coconut milk, cardamom, and cinnamon stick are added. Cook for about 45 to 60 minutes and add some broth if necessary.
3. In the meantime, preheat the oven to 425 °. Peel and chop the potatoes. Bring water to the boil, add the potatoes with turmeric and cook for 5 minutes. Then pour off the water and let it evaporate for about 10 minutes. Spread olive oil together with the potatoes on a baking tray and bake in the oven for 30 minutes.
4. When the potatoes and curry are almost ready, add the coriander, kale, and chicken and cook for five minutes until the chicken is hot.
5. Add parsley to the potatoes and serve with the chicken curry.

Nutrition: Calories: 308.9 Total Fat: 1.4 g Saturated Fat: 0.1 g Polyunsaturated Fat: 0.2 g Monounsaturated Fat: 0.2 g Cholesterol: 72.0 mg Sodium : 1,489.8 mg Potassium: 583.9 mg Total Carbohydrate: 36.1 g Dietary Fiber: 7.7 g Sugars: 4.4 g Protein: 33.0 g

SPINACH AND TURKEY LASAGNA

PREPARATION TIME
30 MINUTES

COOK TIME
25 MINUTES

SERVING
4 PEOPLE

INGREDIENTS

- **9 whole-wheat lasagna noodles**
- **1 teaspoon extra virgin olive oil**
- **½ cup red onion, chopped**
- **1-pound ground turkey breast**
- **3 cups tomato sauce**
- **1/2 cup mushrooms, sliced**
- **1 teaspoon dried parsley**
- **1 teaspoon dried lovage**
- **1 teaspoon dried oregano**
- **¼ teaspoon garlic powder**
- **Salt and pepper to taste**
- **6 cups fresh spinach, chopped**
- **2 cups ricotta cheese**
- **¼ teaspoon ground nutmeg**
- **2 cups shredded mozzarella cheese**

DIRECTIONS

1. If you are trying to cut back on your dairy intake or if you simply find lasagna a bit too rich and cheesy for your preferences, try swapping the ricotta cheese for the crumbled firm or medium-firm tofu. You will be adding another Sirtfood to the dish, and it is much lighter, though surprisingly similar in taste and texture when covered with the sauce.
2. Preheat an oven to 375 degrees F.
3. Bring a large pot of lightly salted water to a boil. Cook lasagna noodles until al dente, approximately 8 minutes. Drain noodles and rinse under cold water.
4. Heat the olive oil in a skillet over medium heat. Stir in the onion and cook until it softens and turns translucent about 2 minutes.
5. Add ground turkey and cook 5 to 7 minutes more, stirring to break up any large chunks of meat.
6. Stir in tomato sauce, mushrooms, parsley, lovage, oregano, black pepper, and garlic powder. Simmer for 2 minutes and season to taste.
7. Combine spinach, ricotta, and nutmeg in a large bowl.
8. To assemble, arrange 3 noodles lengthwise in the bottom of a greased 9x13 inch baking dish. Spread with 1/3 the spinach-ricotta mixture, 1/3 of the turkey mixture, and 1/3 of the mozzarella. Repeat layers, ending with remaining mozzarella.
9. Bake in preheated oven for 25 minutes. Cool for 5 minutes before serving.

Nutrition: Calories: 286.2 kcal Total Fat: 9.6 g Saturated Fat: 4.5 g Cholesterol: 62.1 mg Sodium: 547.3 mg Total Carbs: 31.5 g Fiber: 4.9 g Sugar: 4.1 g Protein: 23.4 g

MEAT

TENDER SPICED LAMB

PREPARATION TIME
5 MINUTES

COOK TIME
40 MINUTES

SERVING
3 PEOPLE

INGREDIENTS

- **1.35kg (3lb) lamb shoulder**
- **3 red onions, sliced**
- **3 cloves of garlic, crushed**
- **1 bird's eye chili, finely chopped**
- **1 tsp turmeric**
- **1 tsp ground cumin**
- **½ tsp ground coriander (cilantro)**
- **¼ tsp ground cinnamon**
- **2 tbsp olive oil**

DIRECTIONS

1. In a bowl, combine the chili, garlic, and spices with a tbsp of olive oil.
2. Coat the lamb with the spice mixture and marinate it for an hour, or overnight if you can.
3. Heat the remaining oil in a pan, add the lamb and brown it for 3-4 minutes on all sides to seal it.
4. Place the lamb in an ovenproof dish. Add in the red onions and cover the dish with foil.
5. Transfer to the oven and roast at 170C/325F for 4 hours.
6. The lamb should be extremely tender and falling off the bone.
7. Serve with rice or couscous, salad or vegetables.

Nutrition: Calories: 166.1 Total Fat: 6.3 g Saturated Fat: 2.2 g Cholesterol: 72.6 mg Sodium: 283.4 mg Potassium: 402.4 mg Total Carbohydrate: 0.9 g Dietary Fiber: 0.0 g Sugars: 0.3 g Protein: 23.9 g

STEAK & MUSHROOM NOODLES

PREPARATION TIME
5 MINUTES

COOK TIME
50 MINUTES

SERVING
2 PEOPLE

INGREDIENTS

- **100g (3½oz) shitake mushrooms, halved, if large**
- **100g (3½oz) chestnut mushrooms, sliced**
- **150g (5oz) udon noodles**
- **75g (3oz) kale, finely chopped**
- **75g (3oz) baby leaf spinach, chopped**
- **2 sirloin steaks**
- **2 tbsp miso paste**
- **2.5cm (1in) piece fresh ginger, finely chopped**
- **2 tbsp olive oil**
- **1-star anise**
- **1 red chili, finely sliced**
- **1 red onion, finely chopped**
- **1 tbsp fresh coriander (cilantro) chopped**
- **1 liter (1½ pints) warm water**

DIRECTIONS

1. Pour the water into a saucepan and add in the miso, star anise, and ginger.
2. Bring it to the boil, reduce the heat, and simmer gently.
3. In the meantime, cook the noodles according to their directions then drain them.
4. Heat the oil in a saucepan, add the steak and cook for around 2-3 minutes on each side (or 1-2 minutes, for rare meat), remove the meat and set aside.
5. Place the mushrooms, spinach, coriander (cilantro), and kale into the miso broth and cook for 5 minutes.
6. In the meantime, heat the remaining oil in a separate pan and fry the chili and onion for 4 minutes, until softened.
7. Serve the noodles into bowls and pour the soup on top.
8. Thinly slice the steaks and add them to the top.
9. Serve immediately.

Nutrition: Calories: 431.1 Total Fat: 14.3 g Saturated Fat: 5.3 g Polyunsaturated Fat: 0.7 g Monounsaturated Fat: 5.2 g Cholesterol: 67.6 mg Sodium   : 311.8 mg Potassium: 195.0 mg Total Carbohydrate: 55.3 g Dietary Fiber: 1.9 g Sugars: 0.3 g Protein: 19.1 g

ROAST LAMB & RED WINE SAUCE

PREPARATION TIME
5 MINUTES

COOK TIME
20 MINUTES

SERVING
3 PEOPLE

INGREDIENTS

- **1.5kg (3lb 6oz) leg of lamb**
- **5 cloves of garlic**
- **6 sprigs of rosemary**
- **3 tbsp parsley**
- **1 tbsp honey**
- **1 tbsp olive oil**
- **½ tsp sea salt**
- **300ml (½ pint) red wine**

DIRECTIONS

1. Place the rosemary, garlic, parsley and salt into a pestle and mortar or small bowl and blend the ingredients.
2. Make small slits in the lamb and press a little of the mixture into each incision.
3. Pour the oil over the meat and cover it with foil.
4. Roast in the oven for around 1 hour 20 minutes.
5. Pour the wine into a small saucepan and stir in the honey.
6. Warm the liquid then reduce the heat and simmer until reduced.
7. Once the lamb is ready, pour the sauce over it, then return it to the oven to cook for another 5 minutes.

Nutrition: Calories: 543 Fat: 37g Carbohydrates: 4g Protein: 35g

SIRTFOOD CAULIFLOWER COUSCOUS & TURKEY STEAK

PREPARATION TIME
5 MINUTES

COOK TIME
45 MINUTES

SERVING
3 PEOPLE

INGREDIENTS

- **150g cauliflower, roughly chopped**
- **1 garlic clove, finely chopped**
- **40g red onion, finely chopped**
- **1 bird's eye chili, finely chopped**
- **1 tsp finely chopped fresh ginger**
- **2 tbsp extra virgin olive oil**
- **2 tsp ground turmeric**
- **30g sun-dried tomatoes, finely chopped**
- **10g parsley**
- **150g turkey steak**
- **1 tsp dried sage**
- **Juice of ½ lemon**
- **1 tbsp capers**

DIRECTIONS

1. Disintegrate the cauliflower using a food processor.
2. Blend in 1-2 pulses until the cauliflower has a breadcrumb-like consistency.
3. In a skillet, fry garlic, chili, ginger, and red onion in 1 tsp olive oil for 2-3 minutes.
4. Throw in the turmeric and cauliflower then cook for another 1-2 minutes.
5. Remove from heat and add the tomatoes and roughly half the parsley.
6. Garnish the turkey steak with sage and dress with oil.
7. In a skillet, over medium heat, fry the turkey steak for 5 minutes, turning occasionally.
8. Once the steak is cooked, add lemon juice, capers, and a dash of water.
9. Stir and serve with the couscous.

Nutrition Calories: 285 Total Carbohydrate: 21.8g Total Fat: 20.0g Protein: 9.6g

TURKEY CURRY

PREPARATION TIME	COOK TIME	SERVING
5 MINUTES	40 MINUTES	3 PEOPLE

INGREDIENTS

- **450g (1lb), turkey breasts, chopped**
- **100g (3½ oz) fresh rocket (arugula) leaves**
- **5 cloves garlic, chopped**
- **3 tsp medium curry powder**
- **2 tsp turmeric powder**
- **2 tbsp fresh coriander (cilantro), finely chopped**
- **2 bird's eye chilies, chopped**
- **2 red onions, chopped**
- **400ml (14fl oz) full-fat coconut milk**
- **2 tbsp olive oil**

DIRECTIONS

1. Heat the olive oil in a saucepan, add the chopped red onions and cook them for around 5 minutes or until soft.
2. Stir in the garlic and the turkey and cook it for 7-8 minutes.
3. Stir in the turmeric, chilies, and curry powder then add the coconut milk and coriander (cilantro).
4. Bring it to the boil, reduce the heat and simmer for around 10 minutes.
5. Scatter the rocket (arugula) onto plates and spoon the curry on top.
6. Serve alongside brown rice.

Nutrition: Calories: 244.8 Total Fat: 7.6 g Saturated Fat: 3.4 g Polyunsaturated Fat: 0.6 g Monounsaturated Fat: 2.0 g Cholesterol: 65.5 mg Sodium : 1,531.1 mg Potassium: 470.9 mg Total Carbohydrate: 19.7 g Dietary Fiber: 2.0 g Sugars: 9.8 g Protein: 24.2 g

FRIED CAULIFLOWER RICE

PREPARATION TIME
55 MINUTES

COOK TIME
10 MINUTES

SERVING
2 PEOPLE

INGREDIENTS

- **1 piece Cauliflower**
- **2 tablespoon Coconut oil**
- **1 piece Red onion**
- **4 cloves Garlic**
- **60 ml (2 fl. oz.) Vegetable broth**
- **1.5 cm (0.60 inch) fresh ginger**
- **1 teaspoon Chili flakes**
- **½ pieces Carrot**
- **½ pieces Red bell pepper**
- **½ pieces Lemon (the juice)**
- **2 tablespoon pumpkin seeds**
- **2 tablespoon fresh coriander**

DIRECTIONS

1. Cut the cauliflower into small rice grains in a food processor.
2. Finely chop the onion, garlic, and ginger, cut the carrot into thin strips, dice the bell pepper and finely chop the herbs.
3. Melt 1 tablespoon of coconut oil in a pan and add half of the onion and garlic to the pan and fry briefly until translucent.
4. Add cauliflower rice and season with salt.
5. Pour in the broth and stir everything until it evaporates, and the cauliflower rice is tender.
6. Take the rice out of the pan and set it aside.
7. Melt the rest of the coconut oil in the pan and add the remaining onions, garlic, ginger, carrots, and peppers.
8. Fry for a few minutes until the vegetables are tender. Season them with a little salt.
9. Add the cauliflower rice again, heat the whole dish, and add the lemon juice.
10. Garnish with pumpkin seeds and coriander before serving.

Nutrition Calories: 230 kcal Protein: 5.13 g Fat: 17.81 g Carbohydrates: 17.25 g

VEGETARIAN CURRY FROM THE CROCK-POT

 **PREPARATION TIME**
6 HOURS 10 MINUTES

 **COOK TIME**
6 HOURS

 **SERVING**
2 PEOPLE

INGREDIENTS

- **4 pieces Carrot**
- **2 pieces Sweet potato**
- **1 piece Onion**
- **3 cloves Garlic**
- **2 tablespoon Curry powder**
- **1 teaspoon Ground caraway (ground)**
- **¼ teaspoon Chili powder**
- **¼ TL Celtic sea salt**
- **1 pinch Cinnamon**
- **100 ml (3 ½ fl. oz.) Vegetable broth**
- **400 g (14 oz.) Tomato cubes (can)**
- **250 g (9 oz.) Sweet peas**
- **2 tablespoon tapioca flou**

DIRECTIONS

1. Roughly chop vegetables and potatoes and press garlic. Halve the sugar snap peas.
2. Put the carrots, sweet potatoes, and onions in the slow cooker.
3. Mix tapioca flour with curry powder, cumin, chili powder, salt, and cinnamon and sprinkle this mixture on the vegetables.
4. Pour the vegetable broth over it.
5. Close the lid of the slow cooker and let it simmer for 6 hours on a low setting.
6. Stir in the tomatoes and sugar snap peas for the last hour.
7. Cauliflower rice is a great addition to this dish.

Nutrition:Calories: 397 kcal Protein: 9.35 g Fat: 6.07 g Carbohydrates: 81.55 g

MEXICAN BELL PEPPER FILLED WITH EGG:

PREPARATION TIME	COOK TIME	SERVING
55 MINUTES	20 MINUTES	2 PEOPLE

INGREDIENTS

- **1 tablespoon Coconut oil**
- **4 pieces Egg**
- **1 piece Tomato**
- **1 pinch Chili flakes**
- **¼ teaspoon Ground cumin**
- **¼ teaspoon Paprika powder**
- **½ pieces Avocado**
- **1 piece green peppers**
- **2 tablespoon fresh coriander**

DIRECTIONS

1. Cut the tomatoes and avocado into cubes and finely chop the fresh coriander.
2. Melt the coconut oil in a pan over medium heat, beat the eggs in the pan, and add the tomato cubes.
3. Keep stirring until the eggs solidify and season with chili, caraway, paprika, pepper, and salt.
4. Finally, add the avocado.
5. Place the egg mixture in the pepper halves and garnish with fresh coriander.

Nutrition Calories: 497 kcal Protein: 20.91 g Fat: 41.27 g Carbohydrates: 14.41 g

FRITTATA WITH SPRING ONIONS AND ASPARAGUS:

PREPARATION TIME	COOK TIME	SERVING
15 MINUTES	30 MINUTES	2 PEOPLE

INGREDIENTS

- **5 pieces Egg**
- **80 ml (3 fl. oz.) Almond milk**
- **2 tablespoon Coconut oil**
- **1 clove Garlic**
- **100 g Asparagus tips**
- **4 pieces Spring onions**
- **1 teaspoon Tarragon**
- **1 pinch Chilli flakes**

DIRECTIONS

1. Preheat the oven to 220°C (430°F).
2. Squeeze the garlic and finely chop the spring onions.
3. Whisk the eggs with the almond milk and season with salt and pepper.
4. Melt 1 tablespoon of coconut oil in a medium-sized cast iron pan and briefly fry the onion and garlic with the asparagus.
5. Remove the vegetables from the pan and melt the remaining coconut oil in the pan.
6. Pour in the egg mixture and half of the entire vegetable.
7. Place the pan in the oven for 15 minutes until the egg has solidified.
8. Then take the pan out of the oven and pour the rest of the egg with the vegetables into the pan.
9. Place the pan in the oven again for 15 minutes until the egg is nice and loose.
10. Sprinkle the tarragon and chili flakes on the dish before serving.

Nutrition Calories: 464 kcal Protein: 24.23 g Fat: 37.84 g Carbohydrates: 7.33 g

VEGETARIAN PALEO RATATOUILLE:

PREPARATION TIME
1 HOURS 10 MINUTES

COOK TIME
55 MINUTES

SERVING
2 PEOPLE

INGREDIENTS

- **200 g (7 oz.) Tomato cubes (can)**
- **½ pieces Onion**
- **2 cloves Garlic**
- **¼ teaspoon dried oregano**
- **¼ TL Chili flakes**
- **2 tablespoon Olive oil**
- **1 piece Eggplant**
- **1 piece Zucchini**
- **1 piece hot peppers**
- **1 teaspoon dried thyme**

DIRECTIONS

1. Preheat the oven to 180°C (350°F) and lightly grease a round or oval shape.
2. Finely chop the onion and garlic.
3. Mix the tomato cubes with garlic, onion, oregano and chili flakes, season with salt and pepper, and put on the bottom of the baking dish.
4. Use a mandolin, a cheese slicer or a sharp knife to cut the eggplant, zucchini and hot pepper into very thin slices.
5. Put the vegetables in a bowl (make circles, start at the edge and work inside).
6. Drizzle the remaining olive oil on the vegetables and sprinkle with thyme, salt, and pepper.
7. Cover the baking dish with a piece of parchment paper and bake in the oven for 45 to 55 minutes.
8. Enjoy it!

Nutrition Calories: 273 kcal Protein: 5.66 g Fat: 14.49 g Carbohydrates: 35.81 g

LENTIL & GREENS SOUP CORN AND BLACK BEAN SOUP

PREPARATION TIME
15 MINUTES

COOK TIME
55 MINUTES

SERVING
6 PEOPLE

INGREDIENTS

- **1 tablespoon olive oil**
- **2 carrots, peeled and chopped**
- **2 celery stalks, chopped**
- **1 medium yellow onion, chopped**
- **3 garlic cloves, minced**
- **1½ teaspoon ground cumin**
- **1 teaspoon ground turmeric**
- **¼ teaspoon red pepper flakes**
- **1 (14½-ounce) can diced tomatoes**
- **1 cup red lentils, rinsed**
- **5½ cups water**
- **2 cups fresh mustard greens, chopped**
- **Salt and ground black pepper, to taste**
- **2 tablespoons fresh lemon juice**

DIRECTIONS

1. Heat olive oil in a large pan over medium heat and sauté the carrots, celery, and onion for about 5–6 minutes.
2. Add the garlic and spices and sauté for about 1 minute.
3. Add the tomatoes and cook for about 2–3 minutes.
4. Stir in the lentils and water and bring to a boil.
5. Now, reduce the heat to low and simmer, covered for about 35 minutes.
6. Stir in greens and cook for about 5 minutes.
7. Stir in salt, black pepper, and lemon juice and remove from the heat.
8. Serve hot.

Nutrition:Calories 174 Total Fat 3.1 g Saturated Fat 0.5 g Cholesterol 0 mg Sodium 59 mg Total Carbs 27.8 g Fiber 12.4 g Sugar 4.8 g Protein 10 g

BUCKWHEAT SPLIT PEA SOUP

PREPARATION TIME
10 MINUTES

COOK TIME
3 HOURS

SERVING
6 PEOPLE

INGREDIENTS

- **1 tablespoon extra virgin olive oil**
- **2 cups dried split peas**
- **½ cup buckwheat groats**
- **1 ½ teaspoons salt**
- **7 cups of water**
- **3 carrots, chopped**
- **3 stalks celery, chopped**
- **1 red onion, diced**
- **3 potatoes, diced**
- **1 teaspoon curry powder**
- **3 cloves garlic, minced**
- **½ cup parsley, chopped**
- **½ teaspoon dried oregano**
- **½ teaspoon dried thyme**
- **½ teaspoon turmeric**
- **½ teaspoon black pepper**

DIRECTIONS

1. In a large pot, sauté the oil, onion, and garlic for 5 minutes on medium heat, or until garlic is fragrant, and the onions are translucent.
2. Add the peas, buckwheat, salt, and water.
3. Bring just to a boil and then reduce the heat to low. Simmer for 2 hours, stirring occasionally.
4. Add the carrots, celery, red onion, potatoes, dried oregano and thyme, turmeric, and ground black pepper. Simmer for another 45 minutes, or until the peas and vegetables are tender.
5. Add the parsley, stir well and allow to steep for a final 10 minutes.

Nutrition: Calories: 165.5 Total Fat: 0.4 g Saturated Fat: 0.1 g Polyunsaturated Fat: 0.2 g Monounsaturated Fat: 0.1 gCholesterol: 0.0 mg Sodium : 75.8 mg Potassium: 781.5 mg Total Carbohydrate: 34.5 gDietary Fiber: 7.9 g Sugars: 3.8 g Protein: 6.8 g

HOT AND SOUR MISO SOUP

PREPARATION TIME
30 MINUTES

COOK TIME
10 MINUTES

SERVING
6 PEOPLE

INGREDIENTS

- **6 dried shiitake mushrooms**
- **2 cups hot water**
- **3 tablespoons soy sauce**
- **5 tablespoons rice vinegar**
- **1/4 cup cornstarch**
- **1 (8 ounces) container firm tofu, cut into 1/4 inch strips**
- **1 (8 ounces) can bamboo shoots, drained**
- **1-quart Miso broth**
- **1/4 teaspoon chili pepper flakes**
- **1 teaspoon ground black pepper**
- **1/2 tablespoon chili oil**
- **1/2 tablespoon sesame oil**
- **1 green onion, sliced**

DIRECTIONS

1. In a small bowl, place shiitake mushrooms in 1 1/2 cups hot water. Soak for 20 minutes, until rehydrated.
2. Drain, reserving the liquid. Trim stems from the mushrooms and cut into thin strips.
3. In a separate small bowl, blend soy sauce, rice vinegar, and 1 tablespoon cornstarch. Place 1/2 the tofu strips into the mixture.
4. In a medium saucepan, mix the reserved mushroom liquid with the vegetable broth. Bring to a boil and stir in the mushrooms and bamboo shoots. Reduce heat, and simmer 3 to 5 minutes. Season with chili peppers and black pepper.
5. In a small bowl, mix remaining cornstarch and remaining water. Stir into the broth mixture until thickened.
6. Mix soy sauce mixture and remaining tofu strips into the saucepan. Return to boil and stir in the chili oil and sesame oil.
7. Garnish with green onion to serve

Nutrition:Carbohydrates: 4 g Sugar: 4 g Fat: 1 g Saturated: 0 g Protein: 1g

GARLIC, SPINACH, AND CHICKPEA SOUP

PREPARATION TIME
10 MINUTES

COOK TIME
25 MINUTES

SERVING
6 PEOPLE

INGREDIENTS

- **2 tablespoons olive oil**
- **4 cloves garlic, peeled and crushed**
- **1 medium yellow onion, coarsely chopped**
- **2 teaspoons ground cumin**
- **2 teaspoons ground coriander**
- **1 1/3 quarts vegetable broth**
- **3 medium potatoes, peeled and chopped**
- **1 (15 ounces) can chickpeas, drained**
- **1 cup heavy cream**
- **2 tablespoons tahini**
- **2 tablespoons cornmeal**
- **3 cups spinach, rinsed and chopped**
- **2 teaspoons fresh parsley, chopped**
- **Chili pepper flakes to taste**
- **Salt to taste**

DIRECTIONS

1. Heat olive oil in a large pot over medium heat and stir in garlic and onion. Cook until tender, 2 – 3 minutes. Season with cumin and coriander.
2. Mix vegetable stock and potatoes into the pot and bring to a boil. Reduce heat and simmer about 10 minutes.
3. Stir in the chickpeas and continue to cook until the potatoes are tender about 5 minutes.
4. In a small bowl, blend the heavy cream, tahini, and cornmeal. Mix into the soup.
5. Stir spinach into the soup. Season with parsley, chili pepper flakes, and salt. Continue to cook until spinach is heated through, about another 5 minutes.

Nutrition: Calories: 389 Fat: 23.5 g Carbohydrates: 39 g Protein: 8.2 g Cholesterol: 54 mg Sodium: 441 mg

CAJUN SHRIMP SOUP

PREPARATION TIME
10 MINUTES

COOK TIME
25 MINUTES

SERVING
6 PEOPLE

INGREDIENTS

- **1 tablespoon extra virgin olive oil**
- **1/2 cup green bell pepper, chopped**
- **1/4 cup green onions, sliced**
- **1 clove garlic, minced**
- **3 cups tomato juice**
- **1 (8 ounces) bottle clam juice**
- **1/2 cup water**
- **1/4 teaspoon dried lovage**
- **1/4 teaspoon dried basil**
- **1/4 teaspoon chili pepper flakes**
- **1 bay leaf**
- **1/2 teaspoon salt**
- **1/2 cup cooked buckwheat groats**
- **3/4 pound fresh shrimp, peeled and deveined**
- **Hot pepper sauce to taste**

DIRECTIONS

1. Warm olive oil in a large pot over medium heat. Sauté bell pepper, onions, and garlic until tender.
2. Stir in tomato juice, clam juice, and water. Season with lovage, basil, chili pepper flakes, bay leaf, and salt.
3. Bring to a boil and stir in buckwheat. Reduce heat and cover. Simmer 15 minutes.
4. Stir in shrimp and cook 5 minutes or until shrimp are opaque.
5. Remove the bay leaf and season with hot sauce to serve.

Nutrition: Calories: 130.9 Total Fat: 3.2 g Saturated Fat: 1.5 g Polyunsaturated Fat: 0.6 g Monounsaturated Fat: 0.7 g Cholesterol: 91.2 mg Sodium: 577.6 mg Potassium: 419.6 mg Total Carbohydrate: 12.5 g Dietary Fiber: 1.7 g Sugars: 4.4 g Protein: 13.4 g

EXOTIC MUESLI WITH TROPICAL FRUITS

PREPARATION TIME
5 MINUTES

COOK TIME
10 MINUTES

SERVING
2 PEOPLE

INGREDIENTS

- **1 small papaya**
- **1 kiwi**
- **1 persimmon not too ripe**
- **100 g coconut muesli (finished product)**
- **200 ml of coconut water (tetra-pack)**

DIRECTIONS

1. Halve the papaya, remove the seeds with a spoon, and peel the papaya. Finely dice the pulp.
2. Peel the kiwi with the peeler and dice the pulp.
3. Wash the persimmon, cut out the stem and dice the pulp. Put the cereal and fruit in bowls and pour the coconut water over them.

Nutrition: Kilocalorie: 280Protein: 14 g Fat: 16 g Carbohydrates: 16 g

SPICY MANGO SALAD WITH SHEEP'S CHEESE

PREPARATION TIME	COOK TIME	SERVING
5 MINUTES	25 MINUTES	1 PEOPLE

INGREDIENTS

- **300 g small, ripe mango (1 small, ripe mango)**
- **4th culms of chives**
- **1 stem**
- **basil**
- **½ organic lemon**
- **pepper from the mill**
- **10 g sheep cheese (9% absolute fat)**

DIRECTIONS

1. Wash the mango, rub dry and peel with a peeler. Cut the flesh from the stone in thick slices, dice, and place in a bowl.
2. Wash herbs and shake dry. Cut the chives into rolls. Pluck the basil leaves, put some aside, and cut the rest into fine strips.
3. Squeeze the lemon, add the juice with chives and basil strips to the mango cubes. Season with pepper and let steep for 10 minutes.
4. Arrange the mango salad. Dab the sheep cheese dry with kitchen paper and crumble it over the salad with your fingers. Garnish with basil leaves.

Nutrition:Kilocalorie: 270 Protein: 18 g Fat: 4 g Carbohydrates: 20 g

CLOUD BREAD

PREPARATION TIME
5 MINUTES

COOK TIME
25 MINUTES

SERVING
9 PEOPLE

INGREDIENTS

- **3 eggs**
- **100 g Cream cheese (Philadelphia type)**
- **1/4 teaspoon baking soda**

DIRECTIONS

1. As a first point, we preheat the oven to 150°C.
2. We separate the whites from the yolks of eggs.
3. We beat the yolks with the cream cheese until obtaining a homogeneous and smooth mass.
4. In a separate bowl, beat the egg whites until stiff with the baking soda.
5. We mix both masses with the help of a spatula, making enveloping movements.
6. We place a sheet of baking paper on a baking sheet, and on it, we distribute 9 piles of dough, forming circles.
7. Bake 20 minutes, the bread cloud or cloud can be made salty (adding rosemary, chopped garlic, salt, pepper or spices) or sweet (adding cocoa). An excellent option is adding york ham or serrano ham.inutes.

Nutrition:Kilocalorie: 230 Protein: 12 g Fat: 15 g Carbohydrates: 10 g

CUCUMBER AND PINEAPPLE SALAD WITH MACKEREL

PREPARATION TIME
5 MINUTES

COOK TIME
20 MINUTES

SERVING
2 PEOPLE

INGREDIENTS

- **Sauce**
- **2 Tablespoons of lime juice**
- **1 Tablespoons fish sauce**
- **1 Tsp cane sugar**
- **2 Tablespoons of rapeseed oil**
- **Salad**
- **2 Spring onions**
- **100 Grams of chicory (red, Treviso, or radicchio salad)**
- **200 Grams of organic cucumber**
- **1 Baby pineapple (330 g)**
- **2 A handful of baby chard (or spinach leaves)**
- **150 Grams of mackerel fillet (smoked, without skin)**
- **40 Grams of peanuts (toasted)**
- **Chilli flakes**

DIRECTIONS

1. For The Sauce. Mix the lime juice, fish sauce, sugar, oil, and 2 tablespoons of hot water.
2. For The Salad. Clean the spring onions, chicory, cucumber, and pineapple or peel if necessary. Cut the spring onions into rings and cut the chicory into fine strips. Dice the cucumber and pineapple 1 cm. Read the chard, rinse it, spin dry. Cut the mackerel into pieces.
3. Mix the spring onions, cucumber, and pineapple with half of the salad dressing. Put the chard and chicory in a flat bowl. First, pour cucumber and pineapple cubes over it, then spread mackerel, peanuts, and chili flakes over it. Drizzle with the remaining salad dressing.

Nutrition:Kilocalorie: 470 Fat: 32g Carbohydrates: 22g Protein: 23g

SALAD WITH EGG, RADICCHIO AND POTATO PASTE

PREPARATION TIME
5 MINUTES

COOK TIME
35 MINUTES

SERVING
2 PEOPLE

INGREDIENTS

- **4 tsp. olive oil**
- **300 Grams of sweet potato (in cubes)**
- **22nd Cloves of garlic (chopped)**
- **1 tsp. spice mix (e.g., "Wilde Hilde" from Herbaria)**
- **2 Organic eggs (hard-boiled, size M)**
- **75 Grams (tomato and pepper in a mild infusion (glass), in pieces)**
- **1 Tablespoons of lemon juice**
- **100 Grams of radicchio (in strips)**
- **3 Spring onions (chopped)**
- **150 Grams of tomato (halved)**
- **40 Grams of green olives (without stone, halved)**
- **2 Tablespoons sunflower seeds (roasted)**

DIRECTIONS

1. Heat a pan, add 3 teaspoons of oil, sweet potatoes, and garlic and stir-fry for about 2 minutes. Pour in 140 ml of water, bring to the boil and cover and simmer for 10-15 minutes. Remove 2 tablespoons of cooking water at the end and mix with the spice mixture. Chop the eggs.
2. Puree the sweet potatoes, tomato peppers and the mixed spice mixture and season the paste with 1 teaspoon of oil and lemon juice.
3. Pour half of the paste into a large screw-top jar and set aside. Spread the other half on a plate, spread half of the salad ingredients and sunflower seeds on top, and sprinkle with the spice mixture if necessary.
4. Fill the cooled paste in the glass as well, chill and eat the next day.

Nutrition:Kilocalorie: 465 Fat: 23g Carbohydrates: 49g Protein: 14g

DESSERT

STRABERRY BUCKWHEAT PANCAKES

PREPARATION TIME
5 MINUTES

COOK TIME
45 MINUTES

SERVING
4 PEOPLE

INGREDIENTS

- **3½ oz. strawberries, chopped**
- **3½ oz. buckwheat flour**
- **1 egg**
- **8fl oz. milk**
- **1 teaspoon olive oil**
- **1 teaspoon olive oil for frying**
- **Freshly squeezed juice of 1 orange**

DIRECTIONS

1. Pour the milk into a bowl and mix in the egg and a teaspoon of olive oil. Sift in the flour to the liquid mixture until smooth and creamy. Allow it to rest for 15 minutes.
2. Heat a little oil in a pan and pour in a quarter of the mixture or to the size you prefer.
3. Sprinkle in a quarter of the strawberries into the batter. Cook for around 2 minutes on each side.
4. Serve hot with a drizzle of orange juice.
5. You could try experimenting with other berries such as blueberries and blackberries.

Nutrition:Calories: 180 kcal Protein: 7.46 g Fat: 7.5 g Carbohydrates: 22.58 g

PANCAKES WITH APPLES AND BLACKCURRANTS

PREPARATION TIME
5 MINUTES

COOK TIME
50 MINUTES

SERVING
2 PEOPLE

INGREDIENTS

- **2 apples, cut into small chunks**
- **2 cups of quick-cooking oats**
- **1 cup flour of your choice**
- **1 tsp baking powder**
- **2 tbsp. Raw sugar, coconut sugar, or 2 tbsp. honey that is warm and easy to distribute**
- **2 egg whites**
- **1 ¼ cups of milk or soy/rice/ coconut**
- **2 tsp extra virgin olive oil**
- **A dash of salt**
- **For the berry topping:**
- **1 cup blackcurrants, washed and stalks removed**
- **3 tbsp. water may useless**
- **2 tbsp. sugar see above for types**

DIRECTIONS

1. As a first point, we preheat the oven to 150°C.
2. We separate the whites from the yolks of eggs.
3. We beat the yolks with the cream cheese until obtaining a homogeneous and smooth mass.
4. In a separate bowl, beat the egg whites until stiff with the baking soda.
5. We mix both masses with the help of a spatula, making enveloping movements.
6. We place a sheet of baking paper on a baking sheet, and on it, we distribute 9 piles of dough, forming circles.
7. Bake 20 minutes, the bread cloud or cloud can be made salty (adding rosemary, chopped garlic, salt, pepper or spices) or sweet (adding cocoa). An excellent option is adding york ham or serrano ham.inutes.

Nutrition Calories: 470 kcal Protein: 11.71 g Fat: 16.83 g Carbohydrates: 79 g

RAW VEGAN WALNUTS PIE CRUST & RAW BROWNIES

PREPARATION TIME
5 MINUTES

COOK TIME
40 MINUTES

SERVING
2 PEOPLE

INGREDIENTS

- **1 ½ cups walnuts**
- **1 cup pitted dates**
- **1 ½ tsp. ground vanilla bean**
- **1/3 cup unsweetened cocoa powder**
- **Topping for Raw Brownies:**
- **1/3 cup walnut butt**

DIRECTIONS

1. Add walnuts to a food processor or blender. Mix until finely ground.
2. Add the vanilla, dates, and cocoa powder to the blender. Mix well and optionally add a couple of drops of water at a time to make the mixture stick together.
3. This is a basic Raw Walnuts Pie Crust recipe.
4. If you need a pie crust, then spread it thinly in a 9-inch disc and add the filling.
5. If you want to make Raw Brownies, then transfer the mixture into a small dish and top with walnut butter.

Nutrition Calories: 899 kcal Protein: 13.83 g Fat: 71.65 g Carbohydrates: 71.67 g

PALEO CHOCOLATE WRAPS WITH FRUITS

PREPARATION TIME
25 MINUTES

COOK TIME
0 MINUTES

SERVING
2 PEOPLE

INGREDIENTS

- **4 pieces Egg**
- **100 ml (3 ½ fl. oz.) Almond milk**
- **2 tablespoons Arrowroot powder**
- **4 tablespoons Chestnut flour**
- **1 tablespoon Olive oil (mild)**
- **2 tablespoons Maple syrup**
- **2 tablespoons Cocoa powder**
- **1 tablespoon Coconut oil**
- **1 piece Banana**
- **2 pieces Kiwi (green)**
- **2 pieces Mandarins**

DIRECTIONS

1. Mix all ingredients (except fruit and coconut oil) into an even dough.
2. Melt some coconut oil in a small pan and pour a quarter of the batter into it.
3. Bake it like a pancake baked on both sides.
4. Place the fruit in a wrap and serve it lukewarm.
5. A wonderfully sweet start to the day!

Nutrition Calories: 555 kcal Protein: 20.09 g Fat: 34.24 g Carbohydrates: 45.62 g

CHOCOLATE GRANOLA

PREPARATION TIME
10 MINUTES

COOK TIME
38 MINUTES

SERVING
8 PEOPLE

INGREDIENTS

- ¼ **cup cacao powder**
- ¼ **cup maple syrup**
- **2 tablespoons coconut oil, melted**
- ½ **teaspoon vanilla extract**
- ⅛ **teaspoon salt**
- **2 cups gluten-free rolled oats**
- ¼ **cup unsweetened coconut flakes**
- **2 tablespoons chia seeds**
- **2 tablespoons unsweetened dark chocolate, chopped finely**

DIRECTIONS

1. Preheat your oven to 300°F and line a medium baking sheet with parchment paper.
2. In a medium pan, add the cacao powder, maple syrup, coconut oil, vanilla extract, and salt, and mix well.
3. Now, place the pan over medium heat and cook for about 2–3 minutes, or until thick and syrupy, stirring continuously.
4. Remove from the heat and set aside.
5. In a large bowl, add the oats, coconut, and chia seeds and mix well.
6. Add the syrup mixture and mix until well combined.
7. Transfer the granola mixture onto a prepared baking sheet and spread in an even layer.
8. Bake for about 35 minutes.
9. Remove from the oven and set aside for about 1 hour.
10. Add the chocolate pieces and stir to combine.
11. Serve immediately.

NutritionCalories: 193 Fat: 9.1 g Carbohydrates: 26.1 g   Protein: 5 g

Days	Breakfast	Lunch	Dinner
1	Kale and blackcurrant smoothie-sirtfood recipes	Coq au vin	Fried cauliflower rice:
2	Green tea smoothie	Kale white bean pork soup	Vegetarian curry from the crockpot:
3	Turmeric chicken & kale salad with honey-lime	Turkey satay skewers	Mexican bell pepper filled with egg:
4	Baked salmon salad with creamy mint	Tomato & goat's cheese pizza	Frittata with spring onions and asparagus:
5	Chocolate cupcakes with matcha icing	Tofu Thai curry	Vegetarian paleo ratatouille:
6	Exotic muesli with tropical fruits	King prawn stir-fry with buckwheat noodles	Strawberry buckwheat pancakes
7	Spicy mango salad with sheep's cheese	Prawn & chili pak choi	Pancakes with apples and blackcurrants
8	Cloud bread	Smoked salmon omelet	Raw vegan walnuts pie crust & raw brownies
9	Cucumber and pineapple salad with mackerel	Mussels in red wine sauce	Paleo chocolate wraps with fruits
10	Salad with egg, radicchio and potato paste	Ginger prawn stir-fry	Chocolate granola
11	Kale walnut bake	Chicken with kale and chili salsa	Kale walnut bake
12	Kale-green bean casserole	Chicken with kale, red onions and chili salsa	Kale-green bean casserole
13	Rice with lemon and arugula	Chicken & bean casserole	Rice with lemon and arugula
14	Cajun turkey stuffing	Chicken curry with potatoes and kale	Cajun turkey stuffing
15	Purple potatoes with onions, mushrooms and capers	Turkey mole tacos	Purple potatoes with onions, mushrooms and capers
16	Corn and black bean soup	Spinach and turkey lasagna	Fried cauliflower rice:

17	Buckwheat split pea soup	Tender spiced lamb	Vegetarian curry from the crockpot:
18	Hot and sour miso soup	Steak & mushroom noodles	Mexican bell pepper filled with egg:
19	Garlic, spinach, and chickpea soup	Roast lamb & red wine sauce	Frittata with spring onions and asparagus:
20	Cajun shrimp soup	Sirtfood cauliflower couscous & turkey steak	Vegetarian paleo ratatouille:
21	Chocolate cupcakes with matcha icing	Turkey curry	Corn and black bean soup

CONCLUSION

Given everything you've heard about the Sirtfood Diet, the most crucial question — at least for a lot of people — is whether it's worth your time and effort.

Some skeptics of this diet, however, argue that these may have been the combined effects of other measurements of weight loss and fitness regimes that those celebrities follow. Most of them have easy access to personal trainers and dietitians, after all.

So, would the Sirtfood Diet still work equally well for an average woman who has relatively limited means?

Multiple studies conducted using animal subjects from a scientific point of view support the claim about the weight loss capabilities of certain sirtfoods, especially blueberries and grapes.

Although the findings of this trial proved quite promising, other experts noted some limitations of the study that could have been improved if subsequent follow-up trials had been carried out.

Some of the most notable limitations identified include:

- Lack of group control to serve as baseline and point of reference;

- Are just 40 participants, a relatively low sample size; and

- Probable bias among participants since they were identified as individuals with health consciousness.

Although not conclusive, these limitations somehow weaken the foundations of the Sirtfood Diet. Some health experts also argue that Sirtfood Diet may help its followers lose weight by enforcing caloric restrictions for a specific time, much like other types of diets.

While restrictive eating can be, to some extent, helpful and useful, several studies have highlighted the negative impacts this practice causes. If you've ever tried to do daily fasting diets, you 'd have encountered mood changes, frequent binges to compensate for lack of food, loss of muscle mass and strength, and even depression.

Given that you won't be expected to perform specific workout workouts or cut down on various types of food, you 'd always need to be mindful of what you're eating and drinking while on the Sirtfood diet. Nonetheless, this amount of leniency that this diet promises to draw a lot of people who don't want to give up a lot of things for a better look and feel.

What, then, is the Sirtfood Diet verdict?

If you're able to live with its drawbacks to reap its rewards and appreciate its rewards over other weight loss programs, then go ahead with your programs to adopt this diet.

Also, most top sirtfoods are fruit, vegetables, and plant-based foods. When combined in your daily meals with the right amount of proteins and carbohydrates, you can't go wrong by eating more of them than you usually do. Just remember to control your red wine, caffeine, and dark chocolate, though, to avoid causing your body unintentionally harm.

Finally, as a rule of thumb, you should not place your 100 percent confidence on a diet that has promised to sound a little too good to be true. Set realistic expectations that are based on your current life situation. Not everybody can live the Sirtfood Diet like Adele and the other celebrities.